HOPING FOR A CURE

ALTERNATIVE CANCER TREATMENT IN MEXICO

Katey Hansen, R.N.

Contents

FOREWORD

At 4:30 p.m., Wednesday, July 19, 2006, my phone rang. It was the call I had patiently been waiting for since having the biopsy.

Hello? Yes, this is Shannon. I'm fine, Nicole, thanks for asking. Oh good, you have my biopsy results. Please say it's good news!

What? Why does the doctor need to tell me the results in person? Is that normal? He wants to see me now?

I lived all the way in the Tahuya Forest, in Mason County, Washington State. At that time of the day, I knew there would be rush hour traffic. I would have to cross the Tacoma Narrows Bridge, and it would be at least a two-hour drive.

I probably wouldn't get to your office until 6:30 or 7:00 p.m. Can I come in tomorrow morning, or could you please ask the doctor to give me my results over the phone?

He wants me to come now? What? Why do I need to bring a support person? Okay.

I hesitated.

Nicole, uh… should I be scared? I don't have a support person to be with me. Okay, fine, I'll just come alone, I'm on my way.

Many who have been diagnosed with cancer can probably relate to much of the phone conversation I had as I received the first hint of my diagnosis. The ride to the doctor's office was terrifying—I cried the entire way, gripping the steering wheel so tightly that my fingers ached. I found it difficult to concentrate on my driving, instead drifting off into fearful thoughts. I think angels must have been steering that day, because I do not recall one moment of that drive. I just remember that when I arrived, all I could see through the

1

glass window was a light shining from the far corner of the medical office. Everything else was dark. It was after hours.

It felt eerie as Nicole escorted me through the dimly lit waiting area to the doctor's private office, instead of the customary examining room. She put a box of Kleenex on his large cherrywood desk, within reach, and handed me a bottle of water decorated with a pink ribbon. My heart sank. This couldn't be good.

That day marked the start of when I found myself transported into a whole new way of life, awkwardly trying to figure out how to win my battle with cancer. I had no idea how to fight against an enemy I had seen do its worst to some of my relatives. I had Stage 3 breast cancer, my life was in danger, and the eleven hundred miles that separated me from my family now felt like an abyss, stretching further into infinity than ever before.

I felt vulnerable and scared. I was a woman thrown into an unfamiliar arena to fight a battle of a magnitude I had never experienced before, and I knew nothing of the enemy. I transformed slowly, and it was painful. I learned that friends and family really cared, and they all had grand ideas as to how I should approach cancer treatment. I felt overwhelmed, because my life depended on my choices. My strategy had to be successful, because I was not willing to die from cancer!

I had a bilateral mastectomy. I was shocked by how I felt afterward. I was not prepared to feel as if I had just gone through an amputation. There had been no discussion, no preparation as to how much loss I would feel after surgery. Breasts are a such a feminine attribute, and I had not realized the emotional pain I would experience once they were gone. I experienced complications from the surgery and became very ill with a staph infection. This complication lent me some time to learn about the world of alternative medicine for cancer.

After surgery, I declined the standard recommended treatments of chemotherapy and radiation. Instead, I went to a small clinic in Arizona. There, I received intravenous vitamin C and B-17, far-infrared sauna, and ultraviolet blood irradiation treatments. About a month later, in May of 2008, testing at the University of Washington revealed that I was in remission. I had beaten Stage 3 cancer, and set out to rebuild my life again. I had reconstructive surgery, but always, in the back of my mind, lingered the very real fear of a recurrence.

I moved back to California in August 2009. It wasn't long afterward until I experienced persistent coughing and pain in my sternum and ribs. In July 2010, I was diagnosed with a recurrence of metastatic breast cancer, which had progressed to Stage 4. The cancer had spread to all lobes of my lungs, my ribs, sternum, and the lymph nodes under my collarbone, as well as other soft tissue areas. My UCLA doctor told my daughter and me that there was no chance of going into remission. The disease, he said, would eventually lead to paralysis, and death. He predicted I likely had only three months to a year to live.

I refused the recommended chemotherapy and hormone blockers, but agreed to forty rounds of radiation to my sternum to slow down the bone metastasis. I completed twenty-two rounds, but had to stop the treatment because of another staph infection and pneumonia. The radiation burned my chest and back, and my lungs. Testing revealed that the cancer had progressed. The radiation therapy had not done any good at all.

After much research and soul searching, I chose CMN Hospital in San Luis Rio Colorado, Mexico. I was admitted in February 2011 for two weeks of advanced alternative cancer treatment. Six months later, I was free of all symptoms. Two months after that, on October 15, 2011, I received the results of my scans. The tests confirmed there was no evidence of disease. The alternative treatments had worked.

Six years later, I am still cancer-free, have learned of healthier ways to heal completely from a diagnosis of cancer, and have devoted my life to sharing what I discovered with others. Many people are learning that we can have hope for a healthier way to recover completely from cancer. I am living proof, and there are many others. You will meet some of them here, in the pages of Katey Hansen's new book, *Hoping for a Cure*.

I was delighted and intrigued when Katey informed me of the book she was writing on her research of both conventional and alternative treatment approaches, and her visits to various alternative clinics in Tijuana. Katey asked

3

if I would read her book and provide her with feedback. I said yes, without hesitation.

We had the first conversation of many that day, and although we have vastly different backgrounds and life experiences, we have much in common. Even though Katey is not a cancer survivor, her professional and personal experiences have made her all too familiar not only with the impact of a cancer diagnosis, but also with the harsh effects of cancer treatment on people's lives.

I found *Hoping for a Cure* to be extraordinary. Katey has shone a light of hope for anyone who wants to choose alternative cancer treatment or integrate alternative medicine in their treatment plan. *Hoping for a Cure* takes us on a journey into the world of alternative cancer treatment, as Katey eloquently shares the stories of the patients she met, her interviews with the doctors, and her descriptions of the various clinics. Many patients who have chosen conventional therapies are told to "get their affairs in order" when the treatment doesn't work. Katey has opened many doors, discovering and investigating clinics and hospitals in Mexico that lead to the real possibility of complete healing of metastatic cancer.

I went to Mexico in order to receive therapies that will likely never be tested in the United States because the drug companies cannot patent natural substances and other non-toxic therapies, many of which Katey describes here, in *Hoping for a Cure*. These include intravenous vitamin C and B17, ozone therapy, ultraviolet light, dendritic cell therapy, autologous bone marrow stem cell therapy—the list of therapies that will not be offered to you by your conventional oncologist goes on and on.

As Katey explains, just because a treatment is not FDA approved does not mean it is ineffective; it simply means the FDA refuses to test it for one reason or another. Contrarily, often the treatment has proven to work and has already been used successfully in Mexico or Germany. I did not get sick with side effects from alternative cancer therapies. I did not vomit or lose my hair, and I was cured in eight months. We are brainwashed to be afraid to leave our country for healing, and into thinking hospitals in Mexico are dirty and dangerous. I saw many hospitals in the United States that were sub-standard, even filthy, when I was a patient. I find that each hospital maintains their own standards, regardless of their location.

My healing was not a miracle. Instead, I feel that managing to survive the barbaric conventional treatments for cancer is what would have been miraculous for me. As Katey will fully explain, chemotherapy and radiation can cause secondary cancers and collateral damage to other parts of our body. Katey also presents research that reveals how chemotherapy often ironically makes cancer more aggressive, promotes metastasis, and causes treatment resistance. The fact that there are not healing therapies made available to help restore a patient's immune system after completing chemotherapy or radiation strikes me as nothing short of cruel and negligent. If a patient chooses conventional treatment, then focusing on the immune system and restoring it should be the other half of their treatment.

Like Katey, I respect the reasons why people accept the therapies recommended by their conventional doctor. Often, a trusting doctor-patient relationship has been established in advance, and that trust plays a role in decision making at a time when the patient is most terrified. A sense of urgency is conveyed by their physician and they respond accordingly, rushing to accept conventional treatment without pausing to discover what other healthier options are available. *Hoping for a Cure* is a valuable resource for those who want to know about these healthier strategies before making treatment decisions.

The patient stories in this book reveal the hard choices that can overwhelm anyone with a diagnosis of cancer. Katey highlights the impact of physiological, psychological, and spiritual factors on our healing. She enlightens us as to how stress and happiness can each impact health. Her dignified approach brings greater understanding of the human spirit and more compassion for those on the cancer journey, regardless of which road to treatment they elect to take. I have never read anything quite like this, and I urge you to read it.

Shannon Knight
Life Coach, Speaker, and Author
Temecula, California
www.shannonknight.com

INTRODUCTION

My good friend Valerie had just been sent home by her doctors to "get her affairs in order," and I arrived at her house not long after, with a healthy dinner and a determination to help her in whatever way I could.

When she answered the door, despite feeling weak and walking with much difficulty, she looked like an African princess in a bright orange and brown jungle-print caftan, and large, dangly gold earrings. Her spirit and loud, contagious laugh had not been weakened by her experience in hospital hell. I don't remember who gave her the nickname "Vivi," but I thought it was so appropriate, given her robust enjoyment of life.

As we sat down to eat, we discussed her plans. Vivi had just had a second surgery for malignant melanoma that had metastasized to the lymph nodes in her leg and pelvis. She refused chemotherapy treatment after being told that it was not usually effective for malignant melanoma. As a former oncology registered nurse like myself, she knew about the suffering the treatment would bring to her life. She wanted to take a different path. Funds were limited and the word "integrative" had not yet come into vogue in the context of medical treatment, much less cancer treatment. She mentioned a television special she had seen some months before that was an "exposé" of a treatment center in Mexico asserting that a special diet and frequent coffee enemas was an effective treatment for cancer. Although intrigued, we laughed at the image of her with her buckets of coffee, lying in weird positions in a seamy clinic in a Third World country, and wondered if snake oil was a part of the treatment too.

You will read more about Valerie, but for now, suffice it to say that I often think back with remorse to that day close to twenty years ago, and question myself about why I didn't research alternative treatment options for one of my best friends. I can only presume that, like many people today, I could not conceive of the idea that hope and potentially effective alternative cancer treatment was available just over the border. I couldn't imagine there was anything better being offered outside the United States, a wealthy country possessing what are considered to be the best hospitals, medical education, research centers, and doctors in the world.

Being a middle-class female in the 1970s, and having a mother who was a nurse, I was pushed by my family to become a nurse as well. My experience with cancer began by default as a new graduate nurse when I was assigned to a GYN/Oncology floor in a major New England hospital. There, I personally administered chemotherapy, without the use of all the protective equipment required today when handling toxic drugs. We didn't even have the intravenous pumps that measure out exact doses of fluids or drugs, and we used the second hand on our watches to count the drips per minute to try to adhere to doctor's orders.

Medical technology has advanced dramatically from those days in the early 1980s, yet the chemotherapy drug Cisplatin I frequently administered is still widely used today for gynecological and other cancers. I have horrible memories of hairless women vomiting and dry-retching, looking so miserable and battered. The only anti-emetic medications available then were quite sedating—likely a good thing. Since those days, there are foods I still can't eat because of some of those memories.

One of my patients, Rachel, did not suffer as much from the chemo-induced nausea and vomiting. Rachel was a woman in her twenties with cervical cancer. She was one of the medical-mistake "DES Daughters" whose mother had been prescribed the medication DES, a synthetic estrogen that was widely prescribed from 1938 to 1971 to help women become pregnant and avoid miscarriage. The female babies born to these women had a very high risk of developing vaginal and cervical cancer at a young age. Though there was no such thing as integrative medicine at that time, Rachel would close her door tightly in the evening, and we were instructed not to enter her room. All the nurses knew to turn a blind eye—and nose—to the fact that

Rachel was smoking marijuana to control the nausea from chemotherapy. Thus, my first exposure to alternative medicine was cannabis, whose therapeutic properties at that time were not as widely known as today, and its medical use was prohibited everywhere in the United States.

I didn't last long working in oncology; the suffering and deaths of my patients were just too much for me to handle. I moved on to working in psychiatry, which used a far more holistic approach, even before the term "holistic" came into vogue.

I really don't know why, but as far back as I can remember I have been interested in alternative medicine and complementary therapies. Possibly, it was because I was raised by a very naturopathic mother, who had a huge organic garden and avoided giving her children medications. Rather than receive vaccines for measles, mumps, or rubella, we were sent to visit other children who had these common illnesses in order to develop immunity at a young age. I don't recall ever being given medication for a fever; the remedies were chicken soup and ginger ale.

Later, as a young adult, I knew at some deep, intuitive level that the body could heal itself if given half a chance. I avoided the burgeoning "better living through chemistry" mindset taking hold in our culture. Over the years, I formally studied homeopathy and herbal medicine, and practiced yoga and meditation, eventually becoming a certified yoga teacher. I began my study of nutrition at age seventeen when I became a vegetarian, despite warnings from the medical science of the day that I would develop a severe protein deficiency and anemia.

Later, I became fascinated with the idea of influencing health and wellbeing through an invisible energy that was well known in Eastern cultures, and began studying and practicing Reiki energy healing. I became a "Reiki Master," an officious-sounding name that meant I had studied and practiced enough to be able to teach Reiki to others. I more recently became very interested in the connection between the mind, spirit, and body and trained to become a Life Coach with Dr. Martha Beck.

Where I live in central North Carolina, we are fortunate to have a cancer support center called Cornucopia House. Complementary therapies such as yoga, massage, and Reiki, as well as education and support groups, are offered to people with cancer, along with their companions and caregivers, free of charge. I began volunteering there, providing Reiki healing sessions and classes to cancer patients and their companions. I was invited to speak about energy healing for the local university hospital's new integrative medicine program, and I raised funds for the center by teaching Reiki classes and energy medicine theory to other health care professionals. I became quite close to some of my clients, and learned through their experiences just how difficult the cancer journey really is. I heard horror stories about the cold and impersonal attitudes of those in the cancer treatment business, as well as heartwarming stories of doctors, nurses, and others displaying great compassion and humanity. I learned how difficult the role of the companion is, and the fear and worry that is their constant companion.

I was, and continue to be, amazed at the bravery, persistence, and resilience of people who are willing to devote their lives to simply being alive and staying alive. My experiences at Cornucopia House and in my own small energy healing/health coaching practice prompted me to develop a passionate interest in not only complementary aids to cancer treatment and recovery but also in the idea that the toxic treatments of chemotherapy and radiation are not our only cancer treatment choices.

Later, my mother taught me so much about the power of the spirit, hope, and a clean diet when faced with cancer. My mom was an adventurous, independent Australian woman who married my father when he was stationed in Australia during World War II. After my father passed away in 1998 from prostate and bone cancer, my eighty-year-old mom wanted to live closer to me, so she moved from New York to North Carolina, with Fluffy, her big white dog, and bought a small house with a large yard so Fluffy would have room to roam. In 2011, at age ninety-two, my mom was healthy and happy, living in her own home, caring for her two cats and a community of deer, squirrels, and birds. (Fluffy had lived to a ripe old age and passed on in 2008.) My mother was a very sociable person who was loved by everyone and had a steady stream of neighbors and friends dropping in, whom she would send home with homemade cookies and rolls, and vegetables from her tiny organic garden.

When my mom began to experience rectal bleeding, it was labeled as hemorrhoids. The cold, stiff-faced gastroenterologist told us that at her age, she was too high a risk for a colonoscopy. He was clearly not interested in helping her, and just went through the motions. A long retired nurse herself, my mother later told me she had known it was cancer, but just didn't want to face it. Six months later, when her symptoms got worse, she was told a flexible sigmoidoscopy could be done with minimal risk. This time she was sent to a far more humane specialist, a compassionate doctor who had tears in her eyes when she told my mom it was indeed colon cancer.

Radiation therapy and the oral chemotherapy drug Xeloda were started. After a couple of weeks, she landed in the hospital due to malaise, lack of appetite, nausea, vomiting, and extreme dehydration, so the radiation therapy had to be paused until she had the strength to show up for daily treatment. I remember a phone call with her radiation oncology nurse shortly after she was discharged from the hospital and before the treatments were resumed, who insisted my mother begin taking Xeloda again. I gently suggested my mother not take it again, at least not until she saw the oncologist, and my typically proper mother agreed, declaring, "I am not taking any of that poisonous chemo crap ever again!" Fortunately, her radiation oncologist advised her against taking any more Xeloda. I hate to think of the more passive and obedient patients who may have listened to that nurse rather than heeding their own common sense and gut feelings.

The radiation therapy did shrink the tumor enough to stop the rectal bleeding, and my mom was faced with the decision of whether or not to have surgery. It seemed so risky for a woman of her age, and I feared the anesthesia would cause dementia, making her unable to live independently. Fully understanding the risks, my mom decided to have the surgery.

Months later, my mom sailed through extensive surgery that included a colostomy, spending about five days in the hospital. She was a favorite among the nursing staff and reminded them when it was time for her to take a walk in the halls—she was determined to avoid pneumonia and blood clots from lying in bed. She confessed she had hoped not to wake up from anesthesia, making her death painless, but since she was alive, she was determined to go back to her independent lifestyle.

A few weeks later we went to see her surgeon for a post-operative check and to discuss the results of the pathology report. The report had surprised her surgeon, as it revealed metastatic ovarian cancer, rather than the primary colon cancer that had seemed evident after the surgery. The surgeon could not conceal his excitement at this unexpected finding, saying her case would have the privilege of being the subject of a presentation for the benefit of other oncologists. Other than the inappropriate eagerness he expressed while my heart was sinking, learning it was metastatic disease, Dr. Calvo proved to be a wonderful doctor, one of those all too rare surgeons who always took his time with patients and had the reputation of never permitting junior doctors to "touch the knife" in the operating room. He had always treated my mom with great care and respect, speaking loudly so she could hear him and patiently answering all her questions. When he recommended that she see a gynecological oncologist, she told him she would not accept chemotherapy. He very kindly asked her to just see the other doctor and hear what she had to say. I did not enthusiastically support my mom's decision to honor Dr. Calvo's request, as I knew what the oncologist would say, but my mother felt she should do what Dr. Calvo asked.

My mom began that appointment by adamantly refusing a pelvic exam, which startled the young GYN/Oncology fellow, but I took this as a good sign that my mom was prepared to take control of the appointment. She told him she did not want chemotherapy and he scurried off to tell the attending oncologist about her refusal of an exam and assertion that she would not accept chemotherapy. When the senior attending doctor arrived, it was clear she was not sure why my mom was even there if she did not want treatment, and I wasn't sure why we were there either. I told her we simply wanted information about what to observe that would indicate progression of disease. The senior doctor replied that my mom had about six months to live and she should go home and enjoy chocolate and wine. I hoped that, due to the oncologist's soft voice, my mom had not heard her issue this death sentence and I quickly changed the subject. While the advice to enjoy chocolate and wine may have been made compassionately, I knew, practically speaking, it could hasten the end of her life, as it is thought by many that cancer thrives on sugar, and although my mom did not drink alcohol, alcohol consumption is known to contribute to cancer risk.

My mom did hear the unsolicited pronouncement of her life expectancy, but she apparently did not take it seriously. She relayed the story of a family friend who lived for many years after being told he only had a year left after a cancer diagnosis, and said she was ready to meet her maker at any time, anyway.

By this time, I had amassed a large library of books and videos about alternative medicine and cancer treatment. My library included titles such as *The Cancer Industry* and *Questioning Chemotherapy*, by Ralph W. Moss, PhD, books about the Gerson Therapy, a nutritional approach to treating cancer, and *Healing Cancer from the Inside Out*, by Mike Anderson, among many others. My mom was a bright woman and an avid reader who had experienced minimal cognitive decline in her later years. Rather than try to influence her decision about the next step and whether or not to try to live, I provided her with books, videos, and articles about nutrition and nontoxic cancer treatment. She decided that she would do her best to live and thrive, using nutrition, and completely changed her eating habits. She purged her kitchen and shopping list of all processed foods, dairy, sweets, and meat. She became an excellent natural foods chef and purchased a juicer. She swapped coffee and black tea for green tea, which she drank throughout the day. And she now treated her frequent visitors, including hospice nurses, to samples of her green juices and vegan fruit-sweetened cookies.

To the surprise of many, not only did she survive, she thrived. She slowly lost the extra weight she had gained in the years prior to the diagnosis and started moving more. Most interesting was that her occasional difficulty with word recall completely disappeared. It seemed that her new lifestyle not only helped her body heal but improved her mental abilities as well. She became a favorite among the hospice nurses, and they gradually reduced the frequency of their visits as my mom continued to thrive and manage her colostomy independently.

Right around her ninety-third birthday, ten months after her last visit with the oncologist, she was discharged from hospice care, against the wishes of her nurses. Her CA-125 (blood marker for ovarian cancer) had dropped down into normal range, and with her lack of symptoms, she was no longer qualified to receive hospice services. My mom bragged that she had been kicked out of hospice, but I knew she missed Jackie, her primary nurse, whose visits were a highlight of her week. By then, my mother had resumed her normal life, driving herself to the grocery store, taking care of her home, and entertaining friends. A kind neighbor planted a vegetable garden for her, so my mother only had to water and harvest.

About a year and a half later, my mom began to decline and told me she was dying, despite normal blood work and no distinct symptoms other than some swelling in her legs. Still mentally sharp, we made plans together for her end of life care and readmission to the in-home hospice program. She grabbed her iPad and said she would have to order new nightgowns and towels if caregivers would be in the house. She instructed me on how to pay her bills and get her house ready for sale after her death. Always concerned about my welfare, we made some changes to her financial affairs that would prevent the estate from having to go through the probate process. We discussed her biggest worry about leaving this world—where her cats would be re-homed.

My mother passed away in 2014, at age ninety-five, at home, with her cats. It is always difficult to lose a parent, at any age, but I take comfort in the fact that her years after cancer diagnosis were enjoyable and not spent in a nursing home, sickened by medical treatments. Although she refused most of the nontoxic supplements I suggested, I believe the change in diet and her decision to embrace the adventure of life a while longer is what allowed her to have another couple of good years.

As I rebounded from the loss of my mother, and the stress of fixing up and selling her house, my work as a psychiatric nurse in a major teaching hospital was becoming increasingly unsatisfying, stressful, and drug focused. I no longer had the time to provide the various educational and yoga groups I had found fulfilling, and much of my workday was spent administering medications and documenting on the increasingly complex computer systems. On my days off, I enjoyed working as a life/health coach, helping women who were trying to recover from various types of physical and mental health challenges. I knew that my true passion was to be somehow involved with a more humane and holistic approach to healing from cancer, and I noticed many people had a huge fear of cancer.

I decided I would leave my full-time job and attempt to fill my days with more inspiring pursuits. Meanwhile, I pondered and prayed for direction toward what might be next. Around this time, the docuseries *The Truth about Cancer* was being broadcast online, and the segments on a couple of the clinics in Mexico reminded me of Valerie and the mystery that shrouded what we knew about treatment in Mexico all those years ago.

Also around this time, my chiropractor casually mentioned that she would not be available for two weeks as she was accompanying her father to Tijuana for the treatment of his recently diagnosed prostate cancer. She told me that many people in her small Midwestern hometown go to this Tijuana physician for everything from Lyme disease to autoimmune disorders to cancer, referred by an integrative physician in the community who is not legally permitted to provide the treatments he believes most effective. I became even more curious about what was going on in Tijuana, and fascinated by people who would refuse or discontinue conventional cancer treatment and travel south of the border armed with trust and hope of a longer or better life. I left my job in January and began researching Mexican clinics and the therapies they offered, and made plans to take the Cancer Control Society bus tour of Mexican clinics that April. But my own brush with the conventional oncology world would delay my trip, yet further propel me toward Mexico.

I went for my yearly visit with my gynecologist, and an ovarian mass was found during the routine exam. I was sent for an ultrasound and initially did not feel too concerned. As the exam proceeded, the young ultrasound technician's demeanor changed from bright and cheerful to very serious, her face masked with concern. I observed her demeanor with alarm, which translated into: "Oh damn, this is not a fibroid!" As it was a Friday, I had to wait, nervously, through the weekend, trying to not think the worst while not denying the possibility that I had cancer. The tension built when I received a call on Monday telling me my doctor needed to see me on Tuesday afternoon and, no, it couldn't be a phone conversation.

When I arrived for my appointment, my visibly upset doctor told me the ultrasound suggested ovarian cancer. I knew that with my family history I was considered to be at a higher risk. I also remembered what I had read some time ago, that many people who are diagnosed with cancer have experienced a major loss or trauma within the previous two years. I had not only lost my mom but had also said goodbye to two of my old and beloved dogs only months after that. Cancer blood markers were drawn, a CT scan was scheduled and I was given a referral to a gynecological surgical oncologist. It was another week before I could see the oncologist and get his interpretation of the CT scan.

I lived with the possibility of an ovarian cancer diagnosis and found myself considering possible treatment options as well as feeling overwhelmed and panicked at the possibility of having to make these decisions. Although I had not heard the dreaded and all too common phrase "You have cancer," I remember living in some sort of dissociative, numb, and other-worldly state, with my future life path completely unknown. I pondered whether it was localized or would the CT scan show that I was Stage IV and full of cancer? I thought there had to be some mistake, as I live a super-healthy lifestyle and help others do the same. The numbing fear and anxiety made the well-intentioned reassurances of my friends hollow and meaningless. I was aware of the poor results achieved by chemotherapy for ovarian cancer, especially if it had metastasized. I knew about the misery of the long- and short-term side effects of chemo and was aware of how chemo can perversely make cancer more aggressive and contribute to metastasis.

I knew that I would not agree to standard treatment.

I searched for the meaning of this experience occurring just as I was getting deep into my research of alternative and integrative cancer treatments. I had crazy thoughts too, thinking I had somehow created cancer in my body from thinking about it too much. I was grateful for my long-time friend Sophie, a gifted healer and Stage III breast cancer survivor who had gone to Germany for integrative treatment many years ago. She did not try to convince me that I did not have cancer; she lovingly helped me to get grounded into my center of peace, where I knew I was OK, no matter what the outcome.

I am extremely grateful that my story has a happy ending as, after surgery a month later, the mass was found to be benign. I certainly don't imply that my experience gave me a true understanding of the emotional roller coaster and suffering that people with cancer endure. However, my experience of being an oncology patient, even briefly, provided a disturbing education about the reality of being a cog on the impersonal cancer industry assembly line. I felt further inspired and motivated to continue my research of not only alternative cancer therapies but the benefits and shortcomings of conventional cancer treatment as well.

With this book, it is my hope that my research, experiences, and the experiences of others I have met along the way will serve to educate and demystify the therapies, clinics, and doctors available across the border and, increasingly, within the United States. I know that seeking alternative or integrative treatment in Mexico or anywhere else will not be for everyone. I hope the information presented about both conventional "mainstream" and alternative treatments will help your decision making, regardless of which path you choose.

My original motivation for writing this book was to offer hope to people with late-stage cancer who have exhausted all treatment options within standard medicine and have been sent home "to get their affairs in order," like Vivi. These people do represent the majority of the patients who seek alternatives in Mexico. But after much research and multiple trips to Tijuana, numerous interviews with patients, and visits to clinics, I was surprised to find many people who were not waiting until they had exhausted all conventional options. Instead, I met many people who had refused standard treatment (especially chemotherapy) from the moment of diagnosis. Others sought treatment in Mexico after they had undergone conventional treatment that was either not proving successful or wasn't tolerable. Some had a recurrence shortly after being declared "cancer free" by their oncologist, and others feared recurrence. Some of their stories will be found in these pages, stories that will answer the question *Who goes to Mexico for cancer treatment, and why?*

Part 1

CHAPTER 1
Bailey's Story

Bailey O'Brien was just twenty years old when she was told she probably only had another six months to live. Bailey had been a healthy, happy, somewhat shy seventeen-year-old, not too much different from her many friends in the Putnam County, New York, community where she grew up. An avid high school athlete, she received a partial scholarship from Boston University and became a promising freshman member of the dive team. Not long into her first semester, she discovered an odd mole on her right temple. She told her mother at the end of Thanksgiving break, and her mother arranged for her to see a dermatologist who did a biopsy of the mole. It was the worst possible news, malignant melanoma. Bailey recounts that she had no idea what to think; she didn't know anything about cancer or melanoma. The day after Christmas, she had her first visit with an oncologist at the nearby Memorial Sloan Kettering Cancer Center, known to be one of the best cancer centers in the country. Bailey had surgery that involved a wide excision of the mole and a sentinel lymph node biopsy. (Sentinel nodes are the first few lymph nodes into which a tumor drains.) As one of the sentinel nodes was found to be malignant, forty-five other nearby nodes were removed. She was now officially diagnosed with Stage III malignant melanoma, one of the most difficult cancers to treat successfully.

She began the recommended interferon treatment, one of the earlier immunotherapies that had become the standard of care for melanoma in the late 1990s. Bailey and her mom were told the interferon had a 50% chance of preventing the cancer from returning, and Bailey resumed her athletics and college life, hoping for the best. Bailey completed the interferon treatment the following May.

Two years later she returned to her oncologist for routine scans, only to find out that the cancer had returned with a vengeance, requiring more surgeries, including one that removed the lower part of her ear. A course of radiation treatment followed the surgeries. Now that the cancer had returned, she was told that the prognosis was even poorer, there was a greater than 50% chance the cancer would return in the next three to five years, and any recurrence would likely progress to terminal disease. Two weeks after completing radiation treatment, while in Hawaii for a training trip with her diving team, she felt a small lump under her chin. She checked with some of her friends to see if they had the same lump as a part of their normal anatomy and her heart sank when she found that they did not.

When Bailey returned to New York and visited her oncologist, her worst fear was confirmed—the cancer was back. Not only was the lump under her chin malignant, there were about half a dozen tumors in her neck, spine, and lung, some considered inoperable. Bailey now had Stage IV malignant melanoma. Bailey felt defeated, thinking that everything she had gone through had been for nothing.

Now that Bailey was Stage IV, she had only a 15–20% chance of surviving five years, according to statistics provided by the American Cancer Society. Bailey's oncologist tried to get her into a clinical trial for a promising new melanoma drug, but her cancer type did not have the right mutations to qualify her for the trial. However, Bailey's oncologist wanted her to begin an experimental treatment of a PABA formulation, one of the B vitamins. She told Bailey that a lab technician had accidentally put PABA in a dish with melanoma cells and it was observed that the cancer cells died. Needing some time to consider this recommendation, Bailey recalls looking out over the expansive view of Boston from her dorm room, thinking that there was a whole vast medical world out there, and yet they had nothing promising to offer her.

Bailey and her mom decided to go to Tulsa, Oklahoma, to visit one of the Cancer Treatment Centers of America hospitals. The Cancer Treatment Centers of America are known for incorporating integrative therapies into cancer treatment, and Bailey thought they might have something that would offer more hope than Sloan Kettering had. Bailey described this visit as a huge disappointment, as the oncologist in Tulsa offered the same chemotherapy and radiation as Sloan Kettering, plus surgery to remove those tumors that were operable. The Tulsa oncologist did not have confidence that these treatments would result in a cure or long-term remission, but would merely buy her more time. Bailey declined, not wanting a slow and painful death, or to spend her last days sick from the treatments.

Soon afterward, Bailey began seeing a New York University (NYU) – Langone Medical Center oncologist. Bailey was told that her cancer was aggressive, and her oncologist pressured her to start an oral chemotherapy drug called Temodar. Bailey agreed, as she was afraid to wait too long to take action, and she completed one round. After she experienced some nausea and malaise, she declined further chemotherapy as her plans for seeking alternative treatment were taking shape.

Since the time of Bailey's diagnosis, one of her mother's friends had begun researching alternative treatment options. The friend had helped other people with her knowledge of holistic healing and she believed that Bailey could overcome the cancer. Although Bailey's mom was open to alternative options as a last resort, until this point she had put her faith in conventional medicine. Bailey did not want to continue the chemotherapy, and she and her mother started to seriously consider other, more promising options.

When Bailey and her mom expressed their interest in alternative therapies, Bailey says the oncologist dropped her as a patient. The oncologist's physician's assistant said, "When Bailey is ready to follow the doctor's protocols, you can call us back and the doctor will be happy to see her."

Bailey's mom and her friend presented some alternative options to Bailey, and they chose a clinic in Mexico that offered Coley's fluid, along with other therapies. Coley's is a bacterial immunotherapy, discovered in the late 1890s by Dr. William Coley, an oncologist at New York's Memorial Hospital, which eventually became Memorial Sloan Kettering. This immunotherapy was used successfully to treat various cancers by many oncologists of that era, including by the Mayo brothers of the original Mayo Clinic, in Minnesota. Coley's fluid, or toxin, as it is sometimes called, is a heat-killed bacterial vaccine that creates a fever by tricking the immune system into thinking an infection is present. Because the bacteria are killed, rather than live, there is no possibility of an actual bacterial infection. A strong immune system response is activated, with the various T cells becoming more active against the cancer.

Unfortunately, the excitement over the newly emerging treatment of radiation therapy and the development of new chemotherapy drugs eclipsed any continuing interest in Dr. Coley's treatment. However, a few physicians continued to quietly use it through the 1960s until the medical-political climate made it illegal.

Bailey and her mom spoke with Gar Hildenbrand, president of the Gerson Research Organization in San Diego and a self-educated epidemiologist and cancer researcher who has worked with several Tijuana clinics for over thirty years. Along with his wife, Christeene, he has tirelessly petitioned Congress to allow a clinical trial of Coley's fluids, and in the late 1980s was involved with a project on unconventional cancer therapies that was sponsored by the former Office of Technology Assessment of the U.S. Congress.

Gar told Bailey and her mom that Coley's treatment provided a 60% chance of success of putting her melanoma into remission, and combined with other treatments, as well as the Gerson Therapy, the chance of long-term remission was even greater. The information about alternative treatments and their potential to help her made sense to Bailey, and she believed it was her best shot. Gar worked as a consultant for CHIPSA Hospital in Playas de Tijuana, a beach suburb of Tijuana, Mexico. Taking what Bailey describes as a giant leap of faith, she and her mom decided to give treatment at CHIPSA a try, and began planning for her admission.

After the NYU oncologist dropped her as a patient, Bailey returned to her original oncologist at Sloan Kettering. Bailey's mother had become convinced that she and Bailey needed to take control of treatment, viewing the oncologists as sounding boards, rather than authorities whose permission was required to make treatment choices. Bailey's mom presented the oncologist with two options: monitor and treat Bailey with the contingency that they were going to Mexico for alternative treatment, or don't treat her at all. This oncologist advised them against going to Mexico and informed them of other drug trials that might be available to Bailey, but he did not drop her as his patient, and agreed to see her when she returned from Mexico.

It was not just her oncologist who thought that they were misguided in going to Tijuana for treatment. Friends and family thought Bailey was crazy to leave the United States when her life was on the line. Bailey says the decision was more difficult for her mom, who felt she would be blamed if things didn't turn out well. When I asked Bailey, who was only twenty years old at that time, if she had been scared, she responded, "I was terrified."

Bailey and her mom set out for Mexico the day before Valentine's Day, spending the night in San Diego before they were met the next morning by a young Mexican man who didn't speak English. Bailey and her mom crossed the border in his old Chevy Suburban, and Bailey recounts feeling terrified during the border-crossing formalities. The obvious poverty of Tijuana along the highway to Playas de Tijuana made her feel even more unsettled. When the driver told Bailey and her mom that they had arrived at the clinic, they couldn't make out exactly where the hospital was among the many storefronts, private homes, and office buildings. They were escorted to what appeared to be a large office building. Bailey did not find the building or the tiny room she and her mom shared for the three weeks of treatment to be particularly comfortable, but in contrast to the cold physical surroundings, the staff were warm, lovely people, who were so kind and caring that Bailey felt safe. (CHIPSA was unfortunately known for being somewhat run-down, but since Bailey's visit, CHIPSA has undergone extensive renovations.)

In addition to the Coley's, Bailey was put on a modified version of the Gerson Therapy, a nutrition-based treatment for cancer and other chronic illness developed by the late physician Dr. Max Gerson, which includes numerous vegetable juices each day, a specific diet, and supplements. As an aspect of the Gerson Therapy, several coffee enemas were prescribed each day for detoxification and stimulation of the immune system. Although coffee enemas are frequently the subject of ridicule by conventional oncology, they have a long history of therapeutic use, and at one time they were in the "bible" of standard medicine—the Merck Manual. Coffee enemas cause dilation of the bile ducts, which aids in detoxifying the liver. The powerful antioxidant glutathione is activated, further enhancing the detoxification, immune stimulation, and pain-relieving effects.

Bailey also received intravenous infusions of vitamin C and laetrile for their ability to target and weaken or kill cancer cells. Intravenous vitamin C is a widely used alternative cancer therapy in Mexico, Germany, and the United States, and has been the subject of research world-wide for its many beneficial effects. Laetrile, an extract from apricot pits, is a unique compound that can selectively damage cancer cells, as well as relieve pain, and its use has a long history of dramatic controversy. Laetrile is largely responsible for the establishment of the alternative cancer clinics in Tijuana in the late 1960s, when it was made illegal in the United States. (Laetrile, and its role in the history of the Tijuana clinics, will be discussed in later chapters.)

In addition, Bailey was given an autologous vaccine as a part of her treatment. Autologous vaccines are a type of immunotherapy prepared from the patient's own blood, or sometimes from a malignant tumor removed during surgery. There are a variety of autologous vaccines, including the widely studied dendritic cell vaccines, but Bailey is not sure exactly what type of vaccine she received. These vaccines are prepared by combining the blood or tumor cells with an immune-stimulant that increases the number of T cells in the immune system. They are prepared and cultured in a lab, then administered as an injection, typically subcutaneously, much as insulin is injected by diabetics. Some doctors administer the vaccines intravenously.

Hyperthermia is another common therapy offered at both Mexican and German clinics, and is also sometimes used in the United States alongside chemotherapy and radiation therapy. Cancer cells are more sensitive to the effects of high heat than normal cells, and the increased temperature weakens or kills cancer cells and makes them more vulnerable to other therapies that target cancer cells. Hyperthermia can be administered using high-tech equipment or the lower-tech immersion in hot water. Although hyperthermia in the form of hot water immersion was recommended as an adjunct to Bailey's treatments, she tried it once and found it intolerably uncomfortable and did not continue the treatment. (CHIPSA now uses modern hyperthermia equipment, rather than hot water immersion.)

While receiving treatment at CHIPSA, Bailey recalls one of the other patients who was very ill with terminal cancer. Bailey was impressed by her positive attitude and lack of fear, despite her poor prognosis. Bailey had never been a religious or even spiritual person, but she began to pray after her terminal diagnosis, asking God for a miracle. After three weeks of treatment, before they left Mexico, it seemed like she had received her miracle. The lump under Bailey's chin was gone. For the next three weeks, at home, Bailey continued elements of the CHIPSA treatment regimen with her mother's help. Her mom gave her injections of the Coley's and the autologous vaccines, and she continued the Gerson dietary program, as well as the coffee enemas.

The day before her twenty-first birthday, Bailey went to her oncologist at Sloan Kettering for scans, about six weeks after her previous visit. Bailey describes a tense and odd series of events that took place immediately following the scans. First, a medical student entered the room and interviewed her about what had taken place in Mexico. Next, some sort of medical assistant entered and asked similar questions. Finally, her oncologist came into the consult room with a blank face. He walked around the room, asking for details about her diet and the therapies she had undertaken in Mexico. Bailey describes feeling confused by his atypical demeanor, and was thinking: *Tell me what is going on!*

Finally, she cried, "What did the scans show?" Expressionless, the oncologist replied, "It appears from the scans there is no sign of active disease." The doctor also said that he was happy for her, and for Bailey to keep doing whatever she had been doing.

Bailey says it was the most emotional moment of her life. A huge weight had been lifted off her shoulders and she cried with joy for days after being pronounced cancer-free. She recounts feeling immensely grateful to have her health back and be given a second chance at life.

Bailey is now twenty-seven years old and has been healthy, with no recurrence of cancer, for seven years. She has discontinued the Coley's she had been self-administering the first few years to keep her immune system tuned up. She follows a less stringent dietary program now, but continues to consume vegetable juices regularly. Bailey says that her experience with cancer and being given another chance has changed her outlook on life for the better. She is now active in a church and maintains a daily spiritual practice. Bailey did much reflection on her life and attitudes before the diagnosis, and now she says she does not want to go a day without living with purpose and intention. She has the steadfast belief that her emotions and thoughts contribute to her health and quality of life. Although Bailey feared a cancer recurrence for a while, she says that her faith in Jesus and her knowledge of, and experience with, the self-healing capabilities of the body has since eliminated this fear.

Bailey finished her undergraduate degree in nutrition and rejoined the dive team in her senior year of college. After graduation, she became certified as a health coach through the Institute of Integrative Nutrition. Bailey now devotes her time to helping other people with cancer through her website (https://www.baileyobrien.com) and personalized health and cancer coaching. She is often invited to speak about her experience with cancer and is in the process of writing her memoir.

It is interesting that Bailey's oncologist wanted Bailey to try an unproven and experimental treatment that was the result of a random lab error in a petri dish. Why was administering an unproven therapy considered more acceptable than an immunotherapy that had been used on thousands of patients for over one hundred years? Would this PABA therapy be considered "mainstream" medicine simply because an NYU oncologist thought it was worth a shot? Would this not have been an "experimental" treatment, just as many of the treatments being used in the alternative clinics of Mexico, Germany, and the United States are labeled? Aren't clinical trials experimental and unproven by their very nature? Bailey tried every "mainstream" and "proven" therapy that conventional oncology had to offer, yet she was put into long-term remission, possibly cured, by therapies that are considered by conventional medicine to be unproven and experimental at best, and outright quackery at worst.

The therapies that Bailey had in Mexico are labeled alternative by The National Center for Complementary and Integrative Health, which defines alternative medicine as a therapy that is a non-mainstream practice used in place of conventional medicine. But at one time, Coley's immunotherapy was considered mainstream in the United States, until radiation treatment captured the enthusiasm of the scientific and medical community.

What is an alternative approach to cancer treatment and how does it differ from the mainstream, conventional approach? What are these therapies and how are they different? Is there any proof to show they are effective? Why can't these therapies be made available in the United States?

CHAPTER 2
What Is an Alternative Approach?

The therapies being used by the doctors in the clinics I have visited in Mexico are most definitely an alternative approach to treating cancer compared to what is considered mainstream in the United States. Yet, I don't believe the term "alternative" accurately describes their treatment protocols. Many of the clinics and doctors use an integrative approach—combining mainstream therapies and/or medications with alternative therapies—as well as placing a greater emphasis on nutrition and lifestyle. A better description may be "an integrative, alternative, and comprehensive approach that strives to improve the healthy functioning of the person, while also targeting cancer." For simplicity, I will refer to this model of treating cancer as "A/I" (alternative/integrative), throughout this book.

Evidence-Based Therapies

The term "evidence based" is used in medicine to describe a treatment that has theoretically been proven safe and effective through a placebo-controlled clinical trial—the "gold standard" in medical research. (Later, I will show how the results of these clinical trials are not as reliable as the cancer industry would like us to believe.) These trials enroll large numbers of people with the same disease, and one group receives the study treatment while the other group receives a placebo, some other type of treatment, or, as is most common in cancer drug research, the typical treatment a person would receive outside of a clinical trial, that is, "the standard of care."

Many of the therapies offered by the clinics in Mexico are considered experimental, and are not "evidence based," as they have not been tested in large clinical trials. However, the treatments being used by the doctors in the A/I clinics *are* science based, and have as evidence the years of use by numerous doctors around the world, especially in Europe. Some of them are being used increasingly in A/I clinics in the United States, as legal regulations allow.

In addition, some of the therapies used in the A/I clinics do have an increasing body of evidence, for example, dendritic cell vaccines—an immunotherapy used by almost all the clinics I visited. Dendritic cell vaccines are the subject of extensive research around the world, and are believed to hold promise in the treatment of cancer. Dendritic cells are sometimes referred to as the sentinels, or policemen, of the immune system, notifying other immune cells to the presence of malignant cells that should be eradicated.

PubMed is a service of the U.S. National Library of Medicine that provides free access to a database of indexed citations and abstracts to medical science journal articles. Enter the words "dendritic cell vaccine" and "cancer" on PubMed and you will be given over 5,000 results to access. One of these results is a review published in *Lancet Oncology,* which reported that dendritic-cell-based immunotherapy is safe and can induce anti-tumor activity, even in patients with advanced disease.[1] Although the authors of this review of prior studies said the vaccines were not found to result in a great reduction in tumor size, they improved overall survival. According to the doctors whom I asked about this study, this improvement in survival is due to the vaccine halting or slowing metastasis. Metastasis refers to the spread of one's cancer to other organ systems, and is responsible for cancer's deadly nature.

The only dendritic cell vaccine that is FDA approved is called Provenge, and it is used for men with metastasized prostate cancer that has not responded to hormone therapy. (The FDA, or Food and Drug Administration, is the government agency in the United States that approves drugs and treatments.) To become FDA approved and made available for use by physicians, the vaccine for each specific cancer must go through a separate and lengthy clinical trial process, often taking many years. Most people with cancer do not have the time to wait so long to try a potentially helpful therapy that does not have the harsh side effects of chemotherapy, and many do not qualify for participation in a clinical trial. Although there are studies in progress in the United States to evaluate whether Provenge can help men with less advanced prostate cancer, it is currently not available outside of clinical trials. A newer prostate-specific immunotherapy, called Prostvac, is currently in phase three clinical trials in the United States and worldwide, and has been proven to extend survival and be safe and well tolerated. Men with prostate cancer can receive this promising new therapy in at least one clinic in Tijuana now.

Most of the physicians in the A/I clinics in Mexico use dendritic cell vaccines for many types of cancer. They are in the category of "autologous vaccines," vaccines made from a patient's own blood via a simple blood draw. The blood is sent to a laboratory where it is cultured to create vast numbers of dendritic cells, and after about two weeks, the vaccine is ready to be administered either as an injection or intravenously. These vaccines have no toxicity and only minimal side effects, and after a dose or two is given at the clinic, patients are given a three- or six-month supply to self-administer at home.

Numerous other natural substances, therapies, and even some older, non-patentable medications have been studied for their contribution in killing cancer cells and preventing metastasis. Hyperthermia, as was offered to Bailey, and a mainstay of treatment in the Mexican and German clinics, produces over 32,000 results on PubMed, reflecting the degree of research interest in using hyperthermia for cancer treatment. Using specialized equipment, hyperthermia can be used locally for superficial tumors as well as a whole-body treatment for other cancers. Sometimes enemas are used, which one physician in a popular Tijuana clinic told me is a safe, gentle, and effective way to raise body temperature. Indiba hyperthermia is a newer technology that uses energy from a radio frequency current that passes between two electrodes, used for local hyperthermia. Although young Bailey found the hot water immersion method of hyperthermia intolerable, most people tolerate hyperthermia without difficulty, and with no adverse effects.

Hyperthermia is used in almost all the A/I clinics in Germany and Mexico due to its ability to weaken or kill cancer cells. In the United States, hyperthermia is only FDA approved for very specific circumstances, but this allows it to be used "off label" by physicians in some of the U.S.-based A/I clinics. In conventional oncology, hyperthermia is sometimes used with, or after, chemotherapy and/or radiation treatment. Outside of clinical research, it is used only for those who cannot tolerate, or who have not responded to, chemotherapy and/or radiation alone. In most A/I clinics in Germany and Mexico, hyperthermia is used along with nontoxic substances that target cancer, or with low-dose chemotherapy.

In the U.S. there have been some studies involving hyperthermia, but there is far more research interest in this therapy in Holland and Germany. A study with very promising results was done recently at Duke University, in North Carolina, using superficial hyperthermia combined with chemotherapy for breast cancer. According to Mark Dewhirst, the director of the study, "Hyperthermia makes blood vessels leaky, putting holes in them so drugs can get into the tumor."[2] There are many other cancer centers in the U.S. that are now studying the use of hyperthermia as an adjunct (complementary add-on) to chemotherapy and radiation therapy.

The intravenous vitamin C (IVC) that Bailey and nearly all of the patients at the A/I clinics receive is another therapy that has an evidence base for being safe and effective, and has been the subject of research for adjunctive use in conventional cancer treatment. IVC is considered by some to be a nontoxic chemotherapeutic agent due to its unique actions. Cancer cells absorb large amounts of vitamin C, possibly because they mistake it for glucose, which has a similar molecular shape. Through enzymatic actions in the cancer cell, peroxide is formed which lyses (dissolves) the cancer cell from the inside out. Vitamin C also boosts immunity and inhibits a specific enzyme that tumors use to metastasize. It induces apoptosis (programmed cell death) and reduces pain, as well as improves energy levels and appetite.[3] IVC has been used for decades and has been found to be safe, with minimal side effects that are easily tolerated when managed by a qualified practitioner. There have been several studies that have examined the effects of IVC on chemotherapy and radiation side effects, tumor markers, inflammation, pain and quality of life of cancer patients, with positive results.[4]

Although hyperthermia and intravenous vitamin C are available at some A/I clinics in the U.S., other therapies used in Mexico and Europe are not. Mistletoe, which produces close to 700 results on PubMed and is a common treatment for cancer in Europe, is not FDA approved. Mistletoe has been studied extensively and is thought to act as a regulator of the immune system and have direct anti-tumor activities. It is believed that it stops or slows metastasis and causes cancer cells to revert to a less aggressive form.

One study found that the survival time of cancer patients treated with Iscador, a common brand of mistletoe, was 40% longer for all types of cancer studied.[5] Other studies have found similar survival benefits.[6] Even the National Cancer Institute has positive things to say about mistletoe, reporting that it is one of the most widely studied alternative therapies for cancer and among the most prescribed drugs offered to cancer patients in Switzerland and Germany, with reports of improved survival and/or quality of life being common.[7] Although dilute oral extracts of mistletoe are available in the United States, the potent prescription formulations for injection used in Europe are not.

The benefits of cannabis for cancer are becoming increasingly known among patients and health providers. Many people have asked me if it is available in the A/I clinics in Tijuana. It was not legal or available during my trips to Tijuana, but could possibly be added to the menu of available therapies at a later date. In June of 2017, medical marijuana was legalized in Mexico, although regulations and policies concerning its availability have not yet been established at the time of this writing. Since the laws in the United States are so strict regarding the transportation of medical cannabis, even from one "legal" state to another, it will likely continue to be illegal to bring medical cannabis products back to the United States from Mexico. It remains to be known if a letter by a Mexican doctor that certifies a qualifying condition for medical marijuana eligibility will be honored by the programs in the many states that have legalized it.

Hyperthermia, IVC, and mistletoe are only a few examples of the various therapies that are used not only by Mexican physicians but also by their peers in Europe. These therapies are not herbs, potions, and nostrums pulled out of the air, or cultural folklore; they are recognized as substances that have been effective against cancer and are the subject of international research interest. Most of these therapies cannot be patented and therefore would not profit pharmaceutical companies, so there is no incentive for them to perform large clinical trials. Also, it is not considered ethically acceptable to withhold the standard cancer treatments, such as chemotherapy and radiation, in order to test nontoxic therapies alone.

The National Center of Complementary Integrative Health (NCCIH), part of the U.S. National Institutes of Health, does fund clinical trials of natural products. Yet, in a single sentence on their website, after stating what the high priority areas are for funded research, the NCCIH support of using natural substances for cancer is very clear: *We also will not fund research that tests natural products for the treatment or prevention of cancer.*[8] No further explanation is given.

They just won't? Not even for prevention? Not even for those who have exhausted all conventional treatment options? I can't help but wonder why. Perhaps it involves complex issues that would result in a loss of funding. (See chapter 4, where I discuss the power and influence the large pharmaceutical companies have over the government and our tax dollars, likely a reason that the NCCIH won't touch cancer.)

Some natural substances have been a part of clinical trials, but typically in combination with chemotherapy and radiation. The purpose of using the natural substances alongside chemotherapy and/or radiation is typically to determine whether they might enhance the effects of standard treatment or minimize the toxic side effects.

Curcumin, the most active ingredient in the spice turmeric, which is derived from a member of the ginger family, is a compound that has received tremendous attention for its ability to target cancer cells. A PubMed search for turmeric and cancer produces close to 4,000 results. A paper was published in 2014 that studied the use of curcumin and its effects on cancer cells and cancer stem cells (CSCs), in colorectal cancer.[9] CSCs are the mother cancer cells, resistant to chemotherapy and thought by scientists to be largely responsible for the metastasis of cancer. The study compared the use of curcumin alone, curcumin combined with the chemotherapy drug 5FU, and 5FU alone in their ability to target and kill CSCs in a laboratory setting. Curcumin, when used on its own, outperformed both the drug and the drug in combination with curcumin in reducing CSCs. The authors, who include Ajay Goel, a cancer researcher at Baylor University Medical Center in Dallas, Texas, concluded that curcumin might be a potential therapy for colorectal cancer, and suppress metastasis.

Availability of Other Technology

The ability of Mexican physicians to use promising therapies that are not yet FDA approved is not limited to drugs and medications but includes diagnostic technologies as well. During a recent trip to Tijuana, I had a diagnostic test called an elastogram that is not available for breast cancer screening in the United States. Elastography measures the rigidity of tissue, because malignant tissue possesses a degree of rigidity that differs from benign masses and normal tissue. I first learned of this test from an acquaintance who was a patient of Dr. Muñoz at the San Diego Clinic in Tijuana. Later, I observed the test being performed when I accompanied a patient at the Biomedical Center for her exam.

Dr. Muñoz and a few other doctors in Mexico use this technology, along with ultrasound, to monitor their breast cancer patients, sparing them exposure to frequent doses of radiation. I surveyed the published literature about this technology and discovered there are studies from Europe and Asia that compare elastography/ultrasound to mammography, ultrasound alone, and elastography alone.[10] The combination of ultrasound and elastography outperformed all of them, including mammography, for accuracy, specificity (benign vs. malignant masses), and a lower number of false positives.

Elastography was developed in the United States but is only FDA approved for the monitoring of patients with liver disease, not as a substitute for mammography. Many women, including me, have concerns about the radiation exposure and ongoing debates about the shortcomings and questionable benefits of mammograms. The literature I surveyed concluded that although more studies should be conducted, elastography with ultrasound has the potential to supplant mammograms.

The result of my elastography and ultrasound was rated a zero, completely normal, and I discovered that my doctor in the U.S. was familiar with elastography and very interested in seeing my report.

The "Standard of Care"

In the U.S. and many other countries, such as Canada, Great Britain, and Australia, physicians are limited to practicing medicine within standard protocols referred to as "The Standard of Care." According to oncologist Guy B. Faguet in his book *The War on Cancer: An Anatomy of a Failure, a Blueprint for the Future*, the term "standard of care" is a legal concept that refers to the level of practice that any average, prudent, and reasonable physician would provide under similar circumstances.[11] Dr. Faguet says, "In essence, from a legal standpoint, standard of care is not necessarily the best, most expensive or technologically advanced care available, but one that is considered acceptable and adequate under similar circumstances." He further states that it is standard of care that determines medical practice, and providing treatment that is considered inferior to the norm is deemed unacceptable, unethical, and renders the physician guilty of negligence and malpractice.

Dr. Faguet is a very vocal critic of chemotherapy and expresses his frustration with these issues related to the standard of care. He says, "Withholding any of the many inefficacious [ineffective] treatments commonly used to manage refractory cancers could be construed as negligence and malpractice."[12] A refractory cancer is one that is not responsive to treatment, so even though a patient's oncologist may know that a prescribed treatment will not be helpful and will cause the patient to suffer from toxic side effects, the treatment must be recommended to protect the oncologist from the consequences of deviating from the established standard of care. Such is often the case with chemotherapy. Thus, people with advanced cancers should realize that their oncologist may not be able to give an honest answer to the question "What would you do, Doc?" if the answer did not reflect the accepted standards of care.

Standard of Care as a Barrier to Innovation

Although mainstream oncology is evolving toward a more personalized therapy approach, by using drugs that are not approved within standard cancer treatment protocols, there are many barriers to be overcome. In a 2016 article in *The New York Times*, Columbia University oncologist and author Siddhartha Mukherjee discusses the challenges of this new personalized medicine. He reports that insurance companies will not pay for "off-label" uses of medicine, and most of the pleas to pharmaceutical companies to provide the medicines for free are denied. He says that the innovative oncologists practicing personalized medicine do what they can, "using their wiles not just against cancer but against a system that can resist innovation."[13] So, even if a patient's oncologist is innovative and bold enough to be willing to justify deviating from the standard of care for the good of the patient, it is likely that the patient's insurance company will refuse to cover treatments that could be helpful or more effective.

Doctors Take Risks When Not Adhering to the Standard of Care

Numerous A/I physicians in the U.S. have been harassed by the FDA and state medical boards as a result of their research and practice of treating cancer in an innovative manner. Physicians risk being disciplined, ostracized, or, as Dr. Faguet points out, found guilty of negligence and malpractice. Although these laws are ostensibly designed to protect us, they limit our choices and infantilize us by forcing us to accept what government agencies say is best. Best for whom is the real question, and often it is not what is best for individual patients.

Even worse than official sanction is the risk of doctors being killed for venturing too far away from conventional medicine. As extreme as this sounds, over sixty mysterious deaths of American integrative physicians and other health care providers have been reported over the past two years, most of whom were treating patients in a nontoxic and innovative manner or researching alternative therapies.[14]

These mysterious deaths began on June 19, 2015, when physician Jeffrey

Bradstreet, formerly of Florida, but practicing in Georgia, was found in a river with a gunshot wound to his chest. Although small town officials called it a suicide, private investigators hired by the family concluded it was murder. Just a few days later, two chiropractors, Bruce Hendendal and Baron Holt, were found dead in Florida. A week later, physician Theresa Sievers was murdered in her home and authorities believed she had been targeted. On the same day, physician Jeffrey Whiteside, a pulmonologist known for his successful treatment of lung cancer, disappeared while vacationing with his family in Wisconsin.

The most well-known doctor who died mysteriously during this time was physician Nicholas Gonzalez of New York, who was known for helping even Stage IV pancreatic cancer patients achieve remission using nutrition, supplements, and detoxification. His family has not released the autopsy report, but they have said that he did not die of a myocardial infarction (heart attack), which was what the media initially reported.

The documented deaths continued into 2017, and according to Erin Elizabeth, a journalist who has written about these deaths and interviewed family members of the victims, many holistic doctors have hired bodyguards and some have shut down their practice altogether. Investigations into these mysterious deaths have been ongoing, with many of the victims' family members hiring private investigators, as they believe that government law enforcement agencies have been too quick to label them accidental. An investigator hired by the wife of one of the victims said he believed her husband had been murdered, and that a "setup" was effected by someone with law enforcement or military training.

None of the documented murders and disappearances of integrative practitioners have been Mexican or German, although two of the murders of Americans occurred in Mexico City. Rumors about who might be responsible for these murders have been plentiful, yet unsubstantiated. There are also bloggers who tend to be anti-alternative medicine, who refer to the deceased doctors as quacks, and dispute any possibility of foul play in their deaths. It's likely the truth will never be known.

Doctors Have More Freedom in Mexico and Other Countries

The danger and criminalization of deviating from conventional standards of care is not a factor in Mexico and Germany. Although the Mexican government oversees the medical training and licensing of physicians and health care facilities, it does not attempt to influence and control the clinical judgment of physicians to the degree the U.S. does. Mexican physicians are free to use treatments from around the world which have been successful in treating cancer, and are free to use therapeutic breakthroughs as soon as they are available.

Although there are dedicated physicians and naturopaths treating cancer in the United States with an A/I approach, in order to stay above the law, they are more limited in the therapies they can provide. It is easy to see the caution that A/I clinics in the U.S. use when comparing their websites to those of the Tijuana clinics. U.S. clinics use vague language to describe their treatment approach, without getting too specific about the therapies they offer. In contrast, the Tijuana-based clinics are quite specific about the various immunotherapy vaccines and natural substances they use to treat cancer.

The FDA Is Watching

The FDA has a program that surveys websites and evaluates the language being used to determine if any regulations are being defied. Andrew Weil, MD, a popular author and founder of the first integrative medicine program in the U.S. at the University of Arizona, was targeted by the FDA for language used on his website. In 2009 Dr. Weil received a "Warning Letter" from the FDA in response to his description of a product called Immune Support Formula. Although his website also included the official recommendations for the flu vaccine, his description of the product said it could help maintain a strong defense against the flu. It said that the formula contained astragalus, which "is used traditionally to ward off colds and flu and has been well studied for its antiviral and immunity-enhancing properties." Part of the FDA's warning letter stated: "The FDA has determined that your website offers a product for sale that is intended to diagnose, mitigate, prevent, treat or cure the H1N1 Flu Virus in people. This product has not been approved, cleared, or otherwise authorized by FDA for use in the diagnosis, mitigation, prevention, treatment, or cure of the H1N1 Flu Virus."[15]

There is indeed plenty of published research about the immune-enhancing effects of astragalus, which comes from the root of a plant belonging to the pea family. It has been used in Chinese medicine for hundreds of years, and it was not being suggested as a replacement for the vaccine. If the FDA sends warnings for the complementary use of harmless herbs for the flu, imagine how they might respond if an integrative cancer clinic in the U.S. listed an unapproved yet widely used therapy such as intravenous mistletoe as one of their therapies for cancer.

A Focus on the Tumor Rather than the Host

Mainstream standard cancer treatment and research in the United States focus on tumor shrinkage using well established and accepted protocols for each type of cancer. Typically, there is no explanation as to why a person got cancer, and a common answer to this question is "bad luck." The unique characteristics, lifestyle, and overall health of the person who has the tumor is of little concern. The success of treatment is measured by the degree of tumor shrinkage, referred to as "tumor response," despite the fact that it is well known that tumor response has no correlation with prolongation of life or the potential for metastasis. If no tumor can be detected with the various scans after treatment, a person is determined to be free of active disease.

Although patients may be counseled about the risk of recurrence after treatment, rarely are they told about the almost inevitable survival of at least some cancer cells, in particular the cancer stem cells (discussed more fully in chapter 4). In the case of chemotherapy, the challenge is how to shrink the tumor without causing such severe adverse effects that the patient's life is at risk. The immune system, damaged by chemotherapy, is weakened in its attempts to defend against metastasis and recurrence of the same cancer, or the development of new cancers.

Conventional oncology, despite growing evidence of the anti-cancer benefit of natural substances and lifestyle changes, typically does not acknowledge or counsel patients about these benefits and strategies that do no harm. Nutritional interventions that are commonly known and proven by research to improve health, and in some cases target cancer, are not a part of standard treatment. Most patients are told to eat whatever they like so long as they get enough calories. Sugar-laden, processed food, such as cookies and candies, are considered comfort food and provided in most outpatient chemotherapy or radiation waiting rooms, despite the fact that refined sugar intake is known to contribute to the inflammation associated with a variety of diseases, including cancer.

Also not usually addressed is the inevitable damage to the body from conventional treatment. Most conventional oncologists do not make any recommendations for supplements, foods, and lifestyle changes that could lessen the side effects and harm caused by the treatments. While it is unfair to expect oncologists, who must prioritize keeping up with the latest research and practice in the increasingly complex world of cancer treatment, to be experts in the benefits of nutrition, supplements, and lifestyle modification, I believe they should be sufficiently aware of these benefits to provide educational resources or refer patients to other practitioners who have a greater knowledge of aids to minimize side effects, recover from harsh treatments, and prevent recurrence. There are a few cancer centers and oncologists who have begun this practice, but these referrals are unfortunately still rare, and most insurance policies will not cover the service.

In contrast, alternative and integrative practitioners worldwide do question why a person has cancer, knowing that inherited genetic mutations play a role in only 5–10% of those with cancer, and many of the genetic mutations identified with sophisticated testing are the *effects* of cancer, rather than the cause.[16] Alternative and integrative doctors know that for the majority of patients, there is some reason why the immune system allowed cancer to grow, and they investigate a person's total lifestyle, history, and micronutrient and metabolic status to try to find the root of the problem. In addition to restoring the optimum functioning of all body systems, A/I treatment focuses on eliminating the cancer through the use of therapies that weaken or kill cancer cells and result in tumor reduction. Even better, these therapies have minimal to no toxicity and no serious side effects. Unlike chemotherapy and radiation, A/I treatment does not make the cancer more aggressive, and often improves immune function and overall health and well-being.

The majority of the physicians of the clinics that I visited in Tijuana are not averse to using conventional medications and therapies that are effective, yet do not harm the patient. Even chemotherapy may be used sparingly, typically in very low doses, coupled with hyperthermia or IPT, insulin potentiation therapy. This method of using chemotherapy has been used for many years in Mexico and Germany and is now being used by a growing number of integrative physicians in the United States. Put very simply, hyperthermia and IPT increase the delivery of the chemotherapy drug to cancer cells, while protecting healthy cells from most of chemo's toxic effects. A solution containing only about 10% of a usual dose of chemotherapy is infused for both the hyperthermia and IPT methods. Although there have been critics of this manner of using chemotherapy, saying there is not enough evidence of its effectiveness, the physicians who use it have seen evidence of its effectiveness and low toxicity. Pharmaceutical companies would not be interested in funding studies that would reduce their profits, so there have been few clinical trials to examine low-dose chemotherapy. This is changing, as researchers at Moffitt Cancer Center at the University of Florida are doing a prostate cancer clinical trial on adaptive therapy, a technique that uses lower doses of chemotherapy, and has the promise to increase survival. According to lead researcher, oncologist Robert Gatenby, "It is hard to get people to think of an alternative approach in which less (chemo) therapy might actually be more effective over time."[17]

Most of the physicians in the Tijuana clinics keep up with the new research and developments in conventional oncology and incorporate those findings compatible with their approach. Many of the physicians are very knowledgeable about immunotherapy and are involved with immunotherapy research, with one clinic having its own accredited laboratory to study these therapies. I had a conversation with a woman who was accompanying her husband to Tijuana for treatment of his Stage IV prostate cancer. She was a former pharmaceutical sales rep, and her husband was an integrative physician in New York. As a physician, he was well aware of the limitations of chemotherapy for metastatic disease, as well as its detrimental effects on quality of life. He wanted to try immunotherapy, but it was not available to him in the U.S., outside of clinical trials. And, in addition to not having a guarantee that one will receive the experimental treatment in a clinical trial, the immunotherapy trials often require that the patient has already received standard treatment, or the trial might include chemotherapy with the immunotherapy.

In addition to various immunotherapies, the physicians in the A/I clinics use a variety of therapies that complement one another, and those who treat patients over a longer period of time change therapies as needed, responding to cancer's ever evolving nature. In addition to the standard cancer blood marker tests that are performed in conventional treatment, many A/I physicians use specialized testing such as the RGCC test, commonly referred to as the "Greece Test," as the developer and first laboratory to perform the test were in Greece. This test can determine the sensitivity of an individual's cancer to a panel of nearly fifty natural substances that are known to have specific actions on cancer cells. These include substances such as laetrile, mistletoe, and curcumin, and there are now laboratories worldwide that perform the test. All of the physicians in Tijuana that I interviewed agreed it is the multifaceted approach, rather than one specific therapy, that can create successful results. None of the doctors promised a "cure," and most said they are able to put about 50% of advanced cancer patients into remission and help improve quality of life for others.

Many people believe that cancer treatment in the United States has become significantly more successful in recent years due to media reports about the success of immunotherapy and the new "precision medicine," with its ability to identify and target genetic mutations with new drugs. There are also many people who appear to have been "cured" after early detection and treatment. Many wonder why anyone would ever travel outside the United States for experimental and allegedly unproven therapies, now that cancer treatment has become so advanced in the U.S. and other developed nations. But how helpful have the genetic understandings of cancer and associated new drugs been for those with advanced disease? How many people are able to benefit from immunotherapy? How have the billions of dollars spent on genetic and immunotherapy research helped those with later-stage cancer, those who have recurrences, and those who have been sent home "to get their affairs in order"?

CHAPTER 3

Media Hype and Theories of Cancer Causation

"I'm starting to hear more and more that we are better than I think we really are. We're starting to believe our own bullshit."
Dr. Otis Brawley, chief medical officer, the American Cancer Society

Promises Unfulfilled

In 1998, the Nobel laureate James Watson, who co-discovered the structure of DNA, declared that scientists would cure cancer in two years, using drugs that block tumor blood supplies. The director of the National Cancer Institute at that time called these drugs "the single most exciting thing on the horizon" for the treatment of cancer.[1]

In 2003, the director of the National Cancer Institute, Andrew C. von Eschenbach, wrote an editorial published in the *Journal of the National Medical Association* entitled "NCI Sets Goal of Eliminating Suffering and Death Due to Cancer by 2015." Referring to the genetic understandings of cancer, von Eschenbach declared, "Our increased understanding of cancer biology is enabling us to design interventions to preempt cancer's progression and, ultimately, to prevent suffering and death."[2]

The public is routinely bombarded with news that tremendous progress is being made toward preventing the suffering and death caused by cancer, yet much of it is inflated and based on preliminary research. A 2016 analysis of the superlative terms used in the media to herald new and promising treatments for cancer revealed that half of the drugs described had not received FDA approval.[3]

Some researchers imply that the media hype serves to bolster the financial interests of investors and others in the health care system and create demands for drugs that are not in the best interest of patients. According to Otis Brawley, oncologist and chief medical officer of the American Cancer Society, "We have a lot of patients who spend their families into bankruptcy getting a hyped therapy that [many] know is worthless. Some choose a medicine that has a lot of hype around it and unfortunately lose their chance for a cure."[4]

Progress

How much progress has been made to preempt cancer's progression? Although death rates from cancer in the U.S. have dropped, most of this decrease is attributed to the early detection and treatment of three of the major causes of cancer death: colorectal, breast, and prostate. These particular cancers are those for which early detection has become possible through screening tests, and treatment is often successful when diagnosed early. The drop in deaths from the fourth major cause of cancer deaths—lung cancer— is attributed to the decrease in the prevalence of smoking.[5] Deaths from these four cancers account for almost half of all cancer deaths.[6] Yet the five-year survival rate for most advanced cancers that have metastasized have barely budged since "The War on Cancer" was declared over forty years ago.[7] For those with metastasized breast cancer, only about 25% live five years or more; for colorectal cancer, that number is only about 14%. Liver cancer, although less common than the four major causes of cancer deaths, is on the rise in the United States and has a five-year survival rate of only 2.8% for metastatic disease.[8] Considering these grim statistics, it is no surprise that many people with advanced cancer would consider taking a chance on other treatment options that may be more successful, feeling that they have nothing to lose by refusing the chemotherapy that diminishes quality of life, can make the cancer more aggressive, and in most cases, is merely palliative, rather than curative. Some have great hopes that these outcomes will soon improve, due to the progress being made in developing new treatments based on the study of the genetic causes of cancer, but are these hopes well founded?

Cancer as a Genetic Disease

The ambitious Human Genome Project, begun in 1990 and completed in 2003, gave scientists the ability to read nature's complete genetic blueprint for building a human being. This international research effort to sequence and map all of the genes of humans provided a resource of detailed information about the structure, organization, and function of the complete set of human genes. Francis Collins, the director of the National Human Genome Research Institute, called it a "transformative textbook of medicine, with insights that will give health care providers immense new powers to treat, prevent, and cure disease."[9]

The Human Genome Project and the International Cancer Genome Consortium, launched in 2008, began an era of intense and prolific research into the genetic underpinnings of cancer. All physicians and researchers worldwide now know that cancer is not just one disease, and that each individual cancer is very complex. A single tumor can have cells that have different genetic makeup, often with over a thousand mutations. There are nearly one thousand known cancer-associated genes in humans, and considering that cells typically need two or more mutations in these genes to become cancerous, there could be more than one million different types of cancer.[10]

Cancer cells do have several characteristics in common, regardless of their specific mutations. They have a lack of responsiveness to signals that would prevent them from growing, they evade apoptosis (programmed cell death), and they cause the non-cancerous tissue to provide them a supply of blood. They can camouflage themselves so that the immune system doesn't recognize them as abnormal cells that should be destroyed. They use the blood and lymph fluids to travel within the body to set up far away from the original tumor site. Although all the different cancers have these characteristics, they do all of this in different ways. Some of the newer cancer drugs are designed to target the precise mechanisms common to all cancer, unlike most of the older chemotherapy drugs that are unselectively toxic to all rapidly dividing cells, including healthy cells.

The most current enthusiasm in research, however, is focused on identifying the various genetic mutations within each cancer, and developing drugs to target them, although the challenges of this genetic approach are enormous. Trying to defeat the multitude of diseases called cancer by identifying all the different mutations and targets and then developing drugs to address the identified unique characteristic of every type of cancer cell is like going on a wild goose chase. Complicating this process is the ability of cancer cells to later develop different mutations and become unresponsive to the drug that targeted the original mutation. This process of targeting genetic mutations has made some significant developments that have helped small numbers of cancer patients, but even those with the identified markers or mutations who qualify for the appropriately matched drug do not always respond. Oncologist Siddhartha Mukherjee, in his book *The Emperor of All Maladies: A Biography of Cancer*, describes targeted therapy as a cat-and-mouse game. He states, "One could direct endless arrows at the Achilles' heel of cancer, but the disease might simply shift its foot, switching one vulnerability for another."[11]

The strategy of identifying genetic mutations, and the drugs that target them, is called "Precision Medicine" or "Targeted Therapy," and although this research is keeping legions of scientists busily employed, it has not yet resulted in successful outcomes for a majority of cancer patients. Although there have been isolated cases of patients having dramatic responses to this approach, according to oncologist Vinay Prasad, "Most people with cancer do not benefit from the precision strategy, nor has this approach been shown to improve outcomes in controlled studies. Precision oncology remains a hypothesis in need of verification."[12] Prasad reported on two studies of patients who were enrolled in genetic sequencing programs that showed only 2–6.4% of patients could be paired with a targeted therapy. He also reported that of the patients with relapsed cancer who have the genetic mutations that can be matched with a drug, only around 30% respond at all, and the median survival is only 5.7 months. He estimates that precision oncology will only benefit about 1.5% of people with solid cancers that have relapsed or have been resistant to other treatments.[13] (Solid cancers are the most common type, and include most all but blood and lymph cancers such as leukemia and lymphoma).

Nobel Prize winner James Watson, whose discoveries paved the way for the gene-centered approach to cancer, was also involved in establishing the Human Genome Project. Watson, now in his late eighties, and considered one of the fathers of molecular biology, has stated that the efforts to locate the genes that cause cancer have been "remarkably unhelpful."[14] Despite the fact that his research laid the foundation for the genetic approach to cancer treatment, he believes that the efforts to sequence DNA to identify mutations and extend life is a "cruel illusion."[15]

Immunotherapy is also considered a very promising strategy within the umbrella term of "precision medicine," and has been the subject of many media reports. Immunotherapy either boosts the body's immune system or trains it in very specific ways to attack cancer cells. There has been enormous enthusiasm for, and investments in, immunotherapy research, with new centers established and philanthropists such as tech billionaire Sean Parker funding many of these centers.

Although some patients have responded dramatically to existing immunotherapies, very few patients benefit from immunotherapy drugs at the present time. In March 2017, oncologists Nathan Gay and Vinay Prasad published the results of their detailed analysis of data, which determined that only 8% of cancer patients may benefit from immunotherapy. Later, in June 2017, Prasad said that there was some new data, and he estimated that number could possibly be as high as 15%.[16] The costs of immunotherapy at present can also be immense, and out of reach for some people who could benefit. The combination of the immunotherapy drugs ipilimumab and nivolumab for the treatment of melanoma results in progression-free survival for nearly one year. This drug combination costs nearly $300,000, and for those with a 20% co-pay, the out-of-pocket cost of $60,000 can be prohibitive.[17]

Combining Prasad's estimates of the number of patients who benefit from immunotherapy with those who are eligible for the genetically matched targeted therapies results in only about 20% of patients who may benefit from these newer therapies. That leaves the other 80% of cancer patients receiving only standard chemotherapy and radiation as the primary treatment after any indicated surgery.

Cancer as a Metabolic Disease

Many scientists argue that cancer is a metabolic disease, rather than a genetic disease. Metabolism refers to the mechanism by which all living things, including every cell, use fuel to create the energy that sustains life. Although these scientists recognize that genetic mutations are found in cancer, the argument is made that cancer is a disease of the mitochondrial energy metabolism, and when this process becomes dysfunctional, the damage to the mitochondria gives rise to genetic mutations. Recall from high school biology that mitochondria are organelles, tiny engines within every cell that create energy in the form of ATP (adenosine triphosphate) and are responsible for cellular respiration.

Thomas Seyfried, a PhD and professor of biology at Boston University, is one of the most outspoken critics of the efforts to identify all the genetic mutations of cancer in the hopes of providing successful treatment. Seyfried labels the prevalent genetic theories of cancer as "dogma" and believes there will not be any major advances in cancer treatment until cancer is recognized as a metabolic disease. Seyfried laments that the findings of the epigenome project caused researchers to go on a misguided search for genetic mutations, and drugs to target them.[18]

Biologist Dominic D'Agostino of the University of South Florida agrees, and believes that the primary drivers of mitochondrial dysfunction are radiation and chemical exposures, various carcinogens, and diet. D'Agostino says that injured mitochondria produce compounds that can damage DNA, and this could explain why most cancers have mutations, as in many cases they are secondary to mitochondrial damage.[19]

The scientists who are proponents of the metabolic theories of cancer causation refer to the research of German physician and scientist Otto Warburg, a 1931 Nobel laureate who first identified the mitochondria of the cell as the central point in the origin of most cancers. Warburg's research revealed that cancer cells are unable to use oxygen properly, and this damaged respiration is the starting point of cancer. Warburg also identified that cancer cells have a unique metabolism, using far more glucose than normal cells and relying on the fermentation of glucose to create energy.

German physician Max Gerson, developer of the Gerson Therapy, also identified mitochondrial dysfunction as the primary driver of cancer. Gerson's theories about the cause of cancer are not as well recognized as those of Warburg, and unlike Warburg, Gerson focused on the balance of potassium and sodium within cells.[20] Prior to Warburg's death in 1970, and the discovery of the first cancer genes in 1971, most scientists viewed cancer as a metabolic disease. The past six years have seen a resurgence of interest in targeting cancer metabolism, with some scientists believing that targeting the metabolic pathways common to all cancer will be a less complex treatment approach than trying to identify a myriad number of genetic mutations.[21]

The research and development of drugs to target the metabolic maladies common to all cancers is underway, with a compound known as 3-bromopyruvate (3BP) receiving the most attention. This compound can block energy production in cancer cells, and the challenges that were involved in its development are the subject of Travis Kristofferson's book *Tripping Over the Truth: The Return of the Metabolic Theory of Cancer Illuminates a New and Hopeful Path to a Cure*. Most of the research pointing to the potential effectiveness of 3BP has been done in the laboratory, with cell cultures or mice. There are two case reports of its successful use in humans that were compassionate uses of 3BP: in a Belgian teenager who had no other options, and a late-stage melanoma patient in Egypt. The Hope4Cancer clinic in Mexico and the Dayspring Cancer Clinic in Arizona have recently begun offering 3BP as one of their therapies. There are many concerns about the safety of 3BP if not administered in a precise manner by someone very familiar with the drug's actions, so research and caution is advised if interested in trying 3BP.

Research has also focused on ways to decrease glucose in the blood, with a new use of the old diabetes drug metformin receiving attention for its ability to influence metabolic pathways. Diabetics taking metformin have been found to be less likely to develop cancer than diabetics who don't take it, and they are less likely to die from cancer if they do get it.[22] The ketogenic diet, discussed in chapter 6, has received a lot of media attention in recent years for its potential to shrink tumors. This dietary strategy severely restricts the carbohydrates that break down into sugar, which is believed to feed cancer cells according to Warburg's theories.

Cancer as a Metabolic AND Genetic Disease

Many cancer researchers now agree that cancer is both a genetic disease and a metabolic disease, in a case of the classic question, "Which came first, the chicken or the egg?" Scientists question whether genetic mutations cause damage to the mitochondria or the damage to the mitochondria causes the genetic mutations. There are researchers working toward identifying genes that affect cancer cell metabolism, as well as those studying the metabolic pathways of cancer and how they affect genetic mutations, in the hopes of interrupting cancer's growth. Of course, cancer is a very complex disease, and the issue of whether it is genetic or metabolic is only one question. The role of the immune system and the environment around and within the tumor are only two of the many factors that influence cancer's growth and spread.

Do Alternative Clinics Treat Cancer as a Metabolic or Genetic Disease?

The cancer treatment programs offered at the A/I (alternative/integrative) clinics in Tijuana have been described as metabolic since a Loyola University biologist, Harold Manner, established a clinic in Tijuana in the early 1980s. Manner coined the term "metabolic therapy" based on his study of the work of John Beard, known for his use of pancreatic enzymes, and that of Ernst Krebs, known for his use of laetrile.

At that time, metabolic therapy was defined as the use of natural food products and vitamins to prevent and treat disease by building a strong immune system. This model focused on the innate self-healing abilities of the human body when it is given the raw materials essential to life and health, rather than a precise and sophisticated focus on the metabolism of cancer cells. Although some of the A/I clinics in Tijuana still refer to their approach as "metabolic," they have added a broader range of therapies than what was available when Manner was alive.

One might question whether any A/I cancer clinics combine alternative therapies with the genetic understandings of cancer. I know of one A/I clinic in the U.S. that uses sophisticated genetic testing as well as alternative modalities, and there may be others. None of the doctors that I spoke with in Tijuana mentioned using genetic testing, or drugs that target genetic mutations, but it is possible that a few of the larger clinics known to use more conventional therapies, along with alternative ones, may be doing so. Considering that most patients who travel to Mexico for cancer treatment have advanced disease, it is likely that they have not had the mutations that qualify them for the few promising targeted therapies, or that all of the treatment options within conventional medicine have been tried and failed to produce remission.

Despite all the media hype about the progress being made with precision medicine, the cancer treatment for most people consists of chemotherapy, as it has for more than sixty years. Why are thousands of cancer patients either refusing or discontinuing chemotherapy and seeking out other treatment options in alternative and integrative clinics in Mexico and Germany, and increasingly within the United States? Is it just that people fear the horrible side effects of chemotherapy that they have seen others endure? Or is it that many of these people have little faith that chemotherapy will improve the quality and quantity of their lives?

CHAPTER 4

Weapons in the War Against Cancer

The May 28, 2001, cover of *Time* magazine pictured a pile of orange capsules, with a headline boldly pronouncing "There Is New Ammunition in the War Against Cancer—These Are the Bullets." Language around the subject of cancer is infused with references to war, especially since the Nixon administration declared war on cancer in 1971. People who have managed to live through grueling cancer treatments are called "survivors," "cancer warriors," and "heroes." They are said to have "beaten" cancer or "won the battle." People who die from cancer have put up "a brave fight" but "lost the battle," implying that, like war, there are winners and losers. Probably the worst use of militaristic language is to label someone with cancer a "cancer victim," or someone who has died of cancer, "a casualty of the war with cancer." It is not surprising, then, that the development of chemotherapy, the most widely used "ammunition" against cancer, has its roots in chemical warfare.

In 1943, Bari, Italy, was a peaceful town of about 65,000 people, blessed with a small but deep harbor hugged by the medieval section of the town. The inhabitants of Bari did not offer any resistance when the British occupied the town during World War II and established it as the main supply center for the British army, as well as the headquarters of the American Fifteenth Air Force division.

On the night of December 2, 1943, about thirty Allied ships were anchored in the small harbor, including the American ship *John Harvey*, with its secret cargo of one hundred tons of mustard gas. On this night, the town was illuminated as usual, and no one anticipated the arrival of a squadron of German bombers delivering an airstrike that would become known as the second Pearl Harbor.

The *John Harvey*, with its toxic load, was one of the fifteen ships sunk that night, but not before exploding and bursting into flames. Although casualties from the airstrike were considered low, given the destruction, many survivors complained of burning sensations, severe eye irritation to the point of blindness, skin rashes, and other unusual symptoms not typically seen in events such as this. At first, the British doctors suspected the Germans had used chemical warfare, but later the truth was revealed.

American physician Stewart Francis Alexander, an expert in chemical warfare, was dispatched to Bari to investigate. Alexander confirmed that the victims had been exposed to chemical weapons, and he traced the mustard gas to the bombs stored on the *John Harvey*. When he reported this to his superiors, he was told to keep silent. There were an unknown number of civilian casualties, estimated at over one thousand, and it was reported that 83 of the 628 military victims died from the chemical exposure.

Alexander returned to the United States with his bags packed full of tissue samples from victims exposed to the mustard gas. It was determined that the gas had decimated the white blood cells within the bone marrow and lymph nodes. Because it was known that, in lymphomas, malignant white blood cells divide uncontrollably, research was undertaken to determine whether the suppressive effects of mustard gas on bone marrow and lymphoid tissue could cure those with lymphoma. Researchers were enthused when the mustard compounds did initially shrink tumors, but similar to the challenges of chemotherapy today, tumors returned and remissions were short-lived.

After World War II and the discovery of the mustard compound's effect on bone marrow, an era of enthusiasm toward using chemical compounds to treat cancer had begun. The next compound to be discovered was aminopterin, a chemical related to folic acid and the predecessor of methotrexate, a cancer drug still in common use that produced remissions in children with acute leukemia. The next twenty years saw a massive effort toward screening natural and synthetic compounds in an effort to determine what other substances could be used as cancer drugs.

In the 1960s, medical oncology did not exist as a clinical specialty, and those who administered chemotherapy were not highly respected, as the main issue of the era was whether cancer drugs caused more harm than good. "Poison" was the general term used for anticancer drugs, and some of the chemotherapists were referred to as lunatics by other physicians.[1] Later in the 1960s, enthusiasm was bolstered by successful treatment of patients with Hodgkin's disease, and in the 1970s, with apparent cures of testicular cancer.

Although chemotherapy has had its share of success in shrinking tumors and extending survival for some patients, Hodgkin's disease, leukemia, and testicular cancer continue to be the few types of cancer for which chemotherapy is considered capable of long-term cures. There are many who question the aggressive use of multiple chemotherapeutic drugs for most of the solid tumor cancers in light of their toxicity, long-term adverse effects, and lack of effectiveness.

The Australian Study

In 2004, a study was published in the Australian journal *Clinical Oncology* titled "The Contribution of Cytotoxic Chemotherapy to 5-year Survival in Adult Malignancies."[2] The term "contribution" refers to the role chemotherapy played among those who survived for five years. For example, according to the American Cancer Society, the overall five-year survival rate of testicular cancer that has spread to nearby lymph nodes is 96% when treated with chemotherapy. According to the findings of this study, for the men who received chemotherapy and survived five years, chemotherapy contributed about 38% to their survival, and something else contributed 62% to their survival. The study was based on an analysis of the results of all the randomized, controlled clinical trials that were done in Australia and the United States between January 1990 and January 2004 that reported a significant increase in five-year survival due to the use of chemotherapy in a variety of adult cancers.

The three authors of this study were all well-respected radiation or medical oncologists in active practice in Australia. The result of their study was that the overall contribution of curative and adjuvant chemotherapy to five-year survival in adults was estimated to be 2.3% in Australia and 2.1% in the United States. According to this study, suffering through nausea, hair loss, infections, and all the other short- and long-term effects of chemo only contributed an average of 2.1% to a person's ability to survive for five years.

These were averages, and the study outlines the different cancers that were a part of the study. These included Hodgkin's disease and testicular cancer with chemo contribution rates of 40.3% and 37.7%, respectively, as well as breast cancer and lung cancer with chemo contribution rates of 1.4% and 2.0%, respectively. The authors reported that they erred on the side of over-estimating the benefit when assumptions were made due to incomplete data. The authors discussed the fact that some of the combination chemotherapy regimens introduced over twenty years ago were still considered to be the "gold standard" of treatment, and stated that the newer regimens have had little impact.

In the concluding discussion the authors wrote, "The introduction of cytotoxic chemotherapy for solid tumours and the establishment of the sub-specialty of medical oncology have been accepted as an advance in cancer management. However, despite the early claims of chemotherapy as the panacea for curing all cancers, the impact of cytotoxic chemotherapy is limited to small subgroups of patients and mostly occurs in the less common malignancies."[3]

In 2006, a commentary of this study was published in *The Australian Prescriber* by Eva Segelov, a medical oncologist in Sydney, Australia. It was titled "The emperor's new clothes – can chemotherapy survive?"[4] Segelov reported that in the medical oncology community there was much outrage and indignation at this "misleading and unhelpful" paper. The study was presented on a popular radio program, and another oncologist, Michael Boyer, then the head of medical oncology at a large Sydney hospital, was invited to provide commentary on the study.

According to Segelov, Boyer raised concerns about the study methodology, saying that he disagreed with the findings and felt the contribution of chemo was higher. Boyer, a respected oncologist, argued that chemo's average contribution to survival was more like 5% or 6%, instead of about 2%—a miniscule difference.[5] This meant that, on average, Boyer attributed 94% to 95% of a person's ability to live for five years, post-diagnosis, to something other than chemotherapy.

According to an article by Ralph Moss, PhD, the Australian study received almost no coverage whatsoever in the United States, calling it an almost total media blackout in North America. Moss closes his article by saying, "Yet nothing can obscure the fact that chemotherapy, for most indications, has far less effectiveness than the public is being led to believe. Dr. Morgan and his colleagues deserve every reader's gratitude for having pointed this out to their colleagues around the world."[6]

I stumbled across the Australian study while researching the effectiveness of chemotherapy for my mother. I had already read the books by Ralph Moss, *Questioning Chemotherapy* and *The Cancer Industry*, and I knew about the lack of effectiveness and high toxicity of chemotherapy, but I admit I was very surprised when I found this indictment published in a well-respected cancer journal. How had I not heard of this study in the United States? Why were these study findings not front page news? Although there have been many papers and articles written by physicians over the years that have questioned chemotherapy, this study likely has the boldest findings. Later, when I discovered the article with the commentary provided by Boyer in an attempt to discredit the study yet acknowledge that chemotherapy contributes only about 6% to survival, I really took notice.

In recent years, the Australian study has been mentioned in books and articles that were written to convince the public that chemotherapy is ineffective. In response, there are numerous rebuttals by those who criticize and ridicule the Australian study, attempting to discredit the study findings. Physician David Gorski, a surgical oncologist and contributor to the website sciencebasedmedicine.org, criticized this study and tore apart its methodology. One of his criticisms was that the study did not include the few cancers that have been most responsive to chemotherapy. Yet, the study did include testicular cancer and Hodgkin's disease, cancers that have become the poster children in the effort to prove how much progress has been made using chemotherapy. The study did not include leukemia, another cancer for which chemotherapy has been effective, as leukemia is treated by hematologists rather than oncologists. In his criticisms, Gorski made no mention of the comments made by oncologist Boyer, who argued against the study's findings, asserting that chemo instead contributed 5–6% to five-year survival rates.

It is difficult to accept that a treatment that produces such quality-of-life-destroying side effects would be recommended and administered as often as it is by physicians if they did not truly believe it was helpful and worth the risks and suffering. I want to believe, as do others, that contemporary medical practice, with its highly educated doctors and modern technology, truly has our best interests in mind. The Australian study was done in 2004, more than twelve years ago at the time of this writing, and I've pondered the question of what findings a similar study would have if performed today. Cancer and cancer drug research is so heavily funded, a contemporary study might show chemotherapy as having a greater contribution to survival than 2%, or even 6%, for the most common types of cancers.

I got an answer when my friend Sha visited me a couple of days after my surgery to remove the ovarian mass they'd found. I hadn't yet received the pathology report, as I didn't want any further surgical intervention at that time and had declined the "quickie" biopsy typically done during a surgery. Sha is a brilliant woman with a PhD in Medical Physics, a full professor at a nearby medical school who has been active in clinical treatment, teaching, and research in the field of radiation therapy for cancer for many years. She has received numerous research grants and traveled the world, teaching and attending conferences in her long career. She has patiently taught me about cancer physiology and her research of using very low-dose radiation to stimulate immune cells to attack cancer cells.

In a conversation about the small possibility that I might have ovarian cancer, Sha revealed that her sister had ovarian cancer, was receiving chemotherapy, and was suffering horrible side effects. Sha casually mentioned that chemotherapy was only about 4–5% effective, so she wasn't holding much hope that chemotherapy would help her sister. My anesthesia-dulled brain perked up at this disclosure, and I said, "Wait, is this your personal opinion, or is it the opinion of the oncologists and other researchers you know?" "Oh, everyone in cancer treatment and research knows this," she replied.

Although by this time I already strongly doubted the effectiveness of chemotherapy in most situations, I found it revealing that all the brilliant scientists and oncologists Sha had known over the years accepted this, while the public seemed to be deluded into thinking of chemotherapy as their best hope of overcoming cancer. I asked myself: If so many professionals in cancer treatment and research know how ineffective chemotherapy is, as the 2004 Australian study suggested, and Sha confirmed in 2016, why is it still being used as the frontline treatment for cancer?

Why Is Chemo Still Frequently Used?

One of the reasons chemotherapy is still used so frequently is that there is little else available that is acceptable within current standards of care. Some of the newer targeted drug therapies and immunotherapies have shown promise for some patients, but as discussed in chapter 3, true therapeutic breakthroughs are rare. "Cut, Poison, and Burn," as the trio of surgery, chemotherapy, and radiation are known, continue to be the predominant treatment choices. Many mainstream, conventional oncologists and cancer researchers have spoken out against chemotherapy, calling it barbaric and expressing their frustration at the slow pace of effective new developments in cancer treatment.

Ulrich Abel, a cancer epidemiologist and biostatistician from Germany, prepared a report back in the early 1990s that presented an analysis of clinical trials and publications that examined the value of chemotherapy in the treatment of advanced epithelial cancer. (Epithelial cancer begins in the cells that line an organ, and is responsible for the most common cancers.) His conclusion was that, with few exceptions, there is no scientific basis for the application of chemotherapy in symptom-free patients with advanced epithelial malignancy.[7]

Oncologist Guy B. Faguet, in his book *The War on Cancer: An Anatomy of Failure, A Blueprint for the Future*, calls the use of ineffective but toxic drugs a model based on flawed premises with an unattainable goal.[8] He believes that cytotoxic chemotherapy in its present form will neither eradicate cancer nor alleviate suffering. In 2005, while other oncologists were lambasting the Australian study, Dr. Faguet made the argument that "only approximately 2% of patients with metastatic cancer treated with chemotherapy will be cured of their disease and prolongation of survival is not feasible for most patients afflicted by most types of cancer."[9]

In his book, Dr. Faguet asserts that the paradigm which viewed cancer as a new growth that is distinct from the person and must be killed at any cost has misguided drug development and patient care for decades. He states that although the explanation as to why this failed system has endured is multifaceted, it can be summarized in one sentence: "The information pipeline, generated by clinical researchers and supported by their sponsors and publishers, fosters standards of care that are reinforced by financial incentives and the extraordinary capacity of physicians for self-delusion, and by unrealistic expectations of consumers nurtured by the media."[10]

Despite their "extraordinary capacity ... for self-delusion," I believe that oncologists would like nothing better than for their patients to get well, and they experience frustration at their limited capacity to effectively treat cancer. Yet, I also feel there are some who are so enmeshed in the system that provides their livelihood that they provide information that presents chemotherapy in far too positive a light, and may leave out facts and information that might influence their patients' decisions about treatment.

An article in *The New England Journal of Medicine* reported that a majority of patients with Stage IV lung and colorectal cancer did not understand that chemotherapy was not at all likely to cure their cancer. Much of the article discusses issues related to how oncologists communicate with their patients, and, curiously, those who gave the highest rating to their doctor were the ones who had an unrealistic expectation of cure from chemotherapy. The authors conclude, "Many patients receiving chemotherapy for incurable cancers may not understand that chemotherapy is unlikely to be curative, which could compromise their ability to make informed treatment decisions that are consonant with their preferences. Physicians may be able to improve patients' understanding, but this may come at the cost of patients' satisfaction with them."[11]

Although the article did not indicate how the less-favored doctors expressed a prognosis, it seems that oncologists could find a way to help a patient have realistic expectations yet not pronounce a death sentence within a specific timeframe, as was given to my mother and many other people with Stage IV cancers. The literature is replete with accounts of patients who have experienced what medical science calls a spontaneous remission, despite a terminal diagnosis.

The stress of a cancer diagnosis can make people more susceptible to suggestion, good or bad. Cell biologist Bruce Lipton, in his book *The Biology of Belief*, describes how our biology adapts to our beliefs, with both our positive and negative beliefs controlling our biology. When our positive beliefs create a positive change in our biology, it is called the placebo effect, but when a negative belief creates a negative change it is called the nocebo effect.[12]

Many have called this nocebo effect "medical hexing," similar to the concept of witch doctors "pointing a bone" at their victims to curse them. Another article in *The New England Journal of Medicine* really drives this point home.[13]

This study of patients who had recently received a cancer diagnosis showed they had increased risks of both suicide and death from cardiovascular causes as compared with the general population. As one might expect, the incidence of both deaths from suicide and cardiovascular causes was highest in those who believed they had a poor prognosis.

One of the most frequent comments I have heard from patients treated for cancer in Mexico concerns the demeanor of the Mexican physicians. They are frequently described as very kind and compassionate doctors who take the time to listen to patients' concerns and answer questions. They are reported to instill hope, yet not sugarcoat the seriousness of the cancer. Some might argue that this is a ploy to obtain and keep patients, but I believe it may be rooted in the Catholic religion and culture of Mexico. A few of the doctors I queried on how they communicate a poor prognosis to patients expressed that only God knows the outcome and "I am not God." They believe in the power of hope in healing, and their culture values the power of prayer. Many of them know from extensive experience that those patients who believe they can get well, and do everything in their power to get well, are the ones who have the best chance of overcoming a serious illness.

"Relative" vs. "Absolute" Survival Benefits

Another way in which chemotherapy can be presented in too positive a light is the way in which statistics and research are reported. This can serve to misinform doctors, patients, and the public alike. The effectiveness of chemotherapy and other treatments is typically presented in relative rather than absolute terms, and this can be very deceptive. Many of the studies, on which oncologists rely to make treatment decisions, and that inform recommendations on whether new drugs should be a part of standard protocols, cite *relative* survival as a percentage. This relative survival percentage is given to the patient to help them make an important decision, yet this information can be deceptive.

If treatment A gives a 1% increase in survival, and treatment B gives a 2% increase in survival, treatment B could then be said to provide a 50% increase in survival over treatment A, despite the fact that treatment B is essentially ineffective. To explain the difference in how this could influence cancer treatment decision making, an example is most illustrative. This fictional example is based on accurate statistical information taken from the website integrativeoncology-essentials.com in an article titled, "The Most Important Statistic You Need to Know," by oncologist Brian D. Lawenda.[14]

Lawenda does not say exactly what stage of breast cancer the statistics refer to, and he uses ten-year survival rates, which are often used when studying breast cancer treatments.

> *Dee has been diagnosed with breast cancer and is unsure if she wants chemotherapy at all, but is willing to have a discussion with her oncologist about the chemotherapy regimens and their chances of improving her ten-year survival. Her oncologist tells her that with chemotherapy, there is a 22.2% improvement in survival compared to no chemotherapy.*

That certainly sounds promising. However, what her oncologist has given her are the RELATIVE survival statistics, not the ABSOLUTE statistics. What this really means is that without chemotherapy she has a 35.8% risk of dying from breast cancer; and with chemotherapy she has a 29.3% risk of dying in ten years.

So, the ABSOLUTE difference is that chemotherapy with a very toxic drug combination would represent a 6.5% improvement in ten-year survival compared to no chemotherapy. Some women may be willing to accept a toxic treatment with only a 6.5% absolute improvement in survival, while others may not be willing, but the point here is that it is impossible to make a fully informed decision without spelling out this information.

> *Dee and her oncologist discuss the two different chemotherapy regimens that are the standard of care in her case. Adriamycin/Taxol is the combination typically prescribed, but Dee knows that Adriamycin is very toxic to the heart and has severe side effects. Her oncologist tells her that the other chemotherapy combination is less toxic but also 2.8% less effective.*

Again, he is stating the RELATIVE difference. Since Dee knows that statistics can be presented in two different ways, she presses her doctor to give her this information in ABSOLUTE terms. The ABSOLUTE difference between the two regimens is only a 0.9% difference in ten-year survival.

Now that Dee knows the ABSOLUTE survival data, she can make a better-informed decision. Chemo with a highly toxic drug gives her only a 0.9% benefit over a more tolerable and less harmful regime, while accepting chemotherapy in any form, with all of its side effects and risks, gives her only a 6.5% improvement in survival.

> *Dee has been researching integrative and alternative treatments, and wonders if an individually prescribed nutrition and supplement regimen, hyperthermia, intravenous vitamin C, immunotherapies, and other nontoxic therapies, including stress reduction and other psycho-spiritual changes, could match or exceed that 6.5%.*

Unfortunately, due to the financial and political realities of clinical trials, there is no definitive data to answer that question. However, I believe that for the thousands of alternative/integrative physicians around the world who are treating cancer with these therapies, the answer would be a resounding YES.

Big Pharma Profits

One of the reasons why chemotherapy continues to be a mainstay of standard cancer treatment is because it creates such huge profits for pharmaceutical companies, and until a greater number of effective immunotherapies and targeted therapies are tested and approved, chemotherapy drugs remain the foundation of the obscenely high profits of "Big Pharma." If there is one subject that both mainstream medicine and alternative/integrative medicine agree on, it is the unscrupulous nature of Big Pharma. Pharmaceutical companies essentially control the treatment of cancer. They exert tremendous influence in every aspect of cancer treatment and research, reaping enormous profits from their involvement in medical education, cancer research, the FDA, major cancer centers, patient interest groups, and the media. They have enormous lobbying power in Washington, D.C., and influence laws and policies for their own benefit.

In her book *The Truth About the Drug Companies: How They Deceive Us and What to Do About It*, physician Marcia Angell, an editor at *The New England Journal of Medicine* for two decades, provides a frightening overview of how Big Pharma exerts its influence. She describes the pharmaceutical industry as "a marketing machine that sells drugs of dubious benefit and uses its wealth and power to co-opt every institution that might stand in its way."[15]

According to Angell, these obstacles include the U.S. Congress, the FDA, academic medical centers, and the medical profession itself. Regarding Big Pharma's influence on medical research, she says that she has seen the pharmaceutical industry influence grow and has become increasingly troubled by the possibility that much published research is seriously flawed. She has seen drug companies exercise a level of control over medical research that was unheard of twenty years ago, with Big Pharma "loading the dice" to make sure their drugs looked good. She believes that flawed research leads doctors to believe new drugs are more effective and safer than they actually are.

In the introduction to his book *Bad Pharma: How Drug Companies Mislead Doctors and Harm Patients,* British physician Ben Goldacre writes, "Drugs are tested by the people who manufacture them, in poorly designed trials, on hopelessly small numbers of weird, unrepresentative patients, and analysed using techniques which are flawed by design, in such a way that they exaggerate the benefits of treatments. Unsurprisingly, these trials tend to produce results that favour the manufacturer."[16]

Goldacre also reports on research that found that pharmaceutical industry-funded trials were about four times more likely to report positive results, and in one case regarding statin drugs, the industry-funded trials were twenty times more likely to give results favoring the test drug.

There is nothing that more sadly illustrates the fact that pharmaceutical companies care only about profits than when one considers that pharmaceutical companies have little interest in developing effective treatments for children with cancer because it is not profitable. According to an ABC News report on this problem, the vast majority of drugs used on pediatric cancer patients were created for adults thirty years ago. With so many different types of pediatric cancers, the market for any particular drug would be small, making it highly unlikely that pharmaceutical companies will take up the cause. Physician Peter Adamson of the Children's Hospital of Philadelphia said, "We are desperate for new treatments. We have not had a single meaningful improvement in pediatric cancer medication in decades and the children have paid the price. Even though we cure four out of five pediatric cancer patients, those who survive often go on to have lifelong side effects from the treatment we give them."[17]

Adverse Effects of Chemotherapy

As it appears that chemotherapy is largely ineffective against most common cancers, and that it contributes little to survival, one might assume that a treatment that carries such great risks and adverse effects would only be used if highly effective, but that is not the case with chemotherapy. Due to the high incidence of cancer, with over 1.6 million new cases diagnosed each year in the U.S. alone, most of us have known someone who has suffered through the immediate toxic effects of chemotherapy.

Since cancer cells rapidly divide, chemotherapy attempts to kill all rapidly dividing cells. Other rapidly dividing cells include those normal cells of the mucous membranes of the mouth, stomach and bowels, hair follicles, and bone marrow. The damage to these tissues is what causes the common chemotherapy side effects of mouth sores, nausea, diarrhea, hair loss, and low blood counts. Damage to bone marrow is responsible for anemia, easy bruising and bleeding, and the impaired ability of the immune system to fight infections. In chapter 6, on nutrition, the importance of healthy gut flora for immune function is discussed, but it should be noted that chemotherapy severely damages this ecosystem, which is an essential contributor to both physical and mental health.

It is well known that chemotherapy reduces circulating lymphocyte levels during and up to three months after treatment. Lymphocytes are a type of white blood cell that is an important part of the immune system. One type of lymphocyte is the B cell, which attacks invading bacteria and viruses. The other types are T cells, which destroy the body's own cells that have become cancerous or infected, and NK (natural killer) cells. NK cells have a unique ability to eliminate cells that have become malignant or infected with viruses. A study published in *Breast Cancer Research* looked at the effects of chemotherapy for breast cancer on immune system health up to nine months post-treatment. Certain types of B and T cells remained significantly depleted even nine months after chemotherapy, and other types showed no sign of returning to pre-chemotherapy levels. The authors found that breast cancer chemotherapy is associated with long-term changes in immune system function.[18]

Some of the other possible side effects of chemotherapy—some temporary, some with chronic, long-lasting effects—include liver, kidney, and heart damage; hearing loss; vision damage; infertility; and cognitive impairment, among many others. Peripheral neuropathy is a common side effect of many commonly used chemotherapy drugs. Peripheral neuropathy is a disorder that affects the nerves that connect the spinal cord to muscles, skin, and internal organs, which can cause weakness, muscle cramps and fatigue, numbness, tingling, and pain. Studies have shown that neuropathy symptoms can occur in 50% of people who have had chemotherapy, continue for two to twelve years after treatment, and have a significant negative effect on quality of life.[19]

Although refinements in dosages and administration techniques have made chemotherapy more tolerable than it has been in the past, and some people are able to weather chemotherapy without serious adverse effects, for others, the treatment is totally debilitating and even life threatening.

Most people survive chemotherapy treatment, but some don't. Infections are typically the cause of death for those who don't make it through chemo, due to the immunosuppressive action of the drugs. Many people have to be admitted to the hospital during the course of chemotherapy treatment, as my mother was, due to infections, dehydration, severe anemia, blood clots, and other life-threatening adverse effects. A friend's mother recently underwent chemo for about three months. In this period of time she required six trips to the emergency room, two 911 calls for assistance, and three hospitalizations for infections and bleeding. The chemotherapy was not effective, and she passed away several months later, while in hospice care.

The late Katie A. Campbell, in her book *The Courage Club*, brings the theoretical knowledge of chemo side effects to life when she describes her experiences after the chemotherapy combination of Adriamycin and Cytoxan for the breast cancer that ended her life far too soon:

> *One morning, about eleven days after my last infusion, I woke up to the reality that I still felt miserably ill. I had been through eleven straight days of pounding headaches, nausea, burning eyes, aching muscles, mouth sores that were inches long and made every bite and sip excruciating, and an overwhelming weakness that had me bent over and shuffling anytime I needed to get up. I realized that I could not bear the thought of going through this for another month.*[20]

The various chemotherapy drugs have different degrees of toxicity and adverse effects, and not everyone has such quality of life disrupting experiences. For some, these side effects may be worth the benefit of tumor shrinkage, and the hope of longer survival. For others, the benefits may not outweigh the risks and the effects on quality of life.

What about Radiation Therapy?

Radiation therapy is typically tolerated more easily than chemotherapy, with fewer immediate and debilitating side effects. Fatigue and skin irritation are the most common, with other side effects contingent on the part of the body that is being irradiated. These can include diarrhea, hair loss, nausea and vomiting, sexuality and fertility issues for both men and women, and pain or burning of the mouth and throat. These short-term side effects usually last a few months after the treatment has stopped.

The technology involved with radiation therapy has been highly refined over the years, with a greatly improved ability to deliver radiation precisely where it is needed, sparing serious damage to nearby tissues. Radiation is very effective at shrinking tumors quickly, and can be invaluable when the location of a tumor threatens life, such as with some brain cancers. My mother got rapid relief of rectal bleeding from radiation therapy, which greatly improved her comfort and quality of life.

It is difficult to estimate the overall contribution of radiation therapy to survival and compare it with that of chemotherapy. The most recent literature examines the effectiveness of radiation therapy on very specific types of cancer. The one study I could find that evaluated the overall survival benefit from radiation therapy was from 1995, and it estimated a survival gain of 16%, excluding skin cancer.[21]

The Susan G. Komen website provides summaries of studies that compare the survival rates of women with Stage II and III breast cancer who received radiation after mastectomy with those who did not. The greatest survival increase, 12%, was found in the ten-year survival rate of women who had had four or more malignant lymph nodes. Other studies have shown only a 3–5% survival benefit from radiation therapy after mastectomy.[22]

Radiation is carcinogenic, and those who have been exposed to radioactive fallout from military operations and nuclear accidents have experienced significantly higher rates of cancer. The most serious adverse effects of radiation therapy, including secondary cancers, can occur later, often many years after treatment. Although radiation can result in rapid tumor shrinkage, it may also contribute to metastasis. Since both chemotherapy and radiation are largely ineffective against cancer stem cells, can contribute to metastasis, and can cause secondary cancers, as well as organ damage, the discussion that follows addresses these issues for the two treatments.

How Chemotherapy and Radiation Fuel Metastasis and Cancer Growth

A major reason for questioning chemotherapy and radiation therapy has to do with their ineffectiveness against cancer stem cells (CSCs). CSCs are tumor-initiating cells that comprise a very small overall percentage of the tumor. CSCs are defined by their unlimited self-renewal ability and their capacity to initiate and maintain malignancy, traits not found in most of the cells that comprise a tumor.[23]

Chemotherapy and radiation are usually successful at shrinking tumors, and are valuable when tumors are life-threatening and must be reduced immediately. However, these treatments do not reduce the chance of metastasis, and may even accelerate the spread to other organs. Metastasizing cancer is what eventually causes people to succumb to the disease, rather than the presence of the initial tumor itself.

Researchers are confounded by the inability of chemotherapy to kill CSCs and, often, multiple highly toxic chemotherapy agents are used in the (usually ineffective) attempts to kill these master cells that can circulate through the body and create more tumors. Radiation treatment and chemotherapy often kill the bulk of cancer cells, but are not able to eliminate the CSCs. The surviving CSCs give rise to new tumors which become more malignant, fast-spreading, and resistant to chemo and radiation, making the prognosis dismal.[24]

Recent research from the Fred Hutchinson Cancer Research Center in

Seattle has identified another mechanism by which chemotherapy fuels cancer growth and metastasis. In their study published in *Nature Medicine*, they described the effect of chemotherapy on healthy connective tissue cells called fibroblasts. When the fibroblasts were exposed to chemotherapy, they secreted a protein called WNT16B into the tumor microenvironment, which promoted tumor cell survival and disease progression. Scientists observed an up to thirty-fold increase in this tumor-promoting protein in response to chemotherapy. The study's authors state that these results outline the way in which toxic therapies, given in a cyclical manner, can create future treatment resistance.[25]

This tumor microenvironment that protects CSCs and has a suppressing effect on the immune system is the subject of current research, especially in the development of drugs that target pathways involved with CSCs. The challenge is that the biology of CSCs may differ among varying cancers, and the protective tumor microenvironment interferes with the drug's penetration into the tumor.[26]

Even more concerning is recent research that suggests chemo can induce tissues in other organs to become more hospitable to cancer cells.

A 2017 study from Ohio State University discovered that the chemo drug paclitaxel (Taxol, Onxal), a front-line chemo drug for breast cancer and used for many other cancers, can fuel the spread of cancer to the lungs and allow breast cancer cells to escape the tumor.[27]

Professor of biological chemistry and pharmacology Tsonwin Hai, the study's senior author, said, "That chemotherapy can paradoxically promote cancer progression is an emerging revelation in cancer research. However, a molecular-level understanding of this devastating effect is not clear." The researchers identified a particular gene that is known to be turned on by stress, and this gene is found to have higher expression in those who had chemotherapy. According to Hai, "This gene seems to do two things at once: essentially help distribute the 'seeds' (cancer cells) and fertilize the 'soil' (the lung)."[28]

Chemotherapy is not the only treatment that can make cancer more aggressive. There are studies that suggest that radiation treatment transforms less aggressive breast cancer cells into more aggressive CSCs. One of these studies found that the breast cancer cells that transformed into CSCs had a more than thirty-fold increased ability to form tumors than non-irradiated breast cancer cells.[29]

Another study, in the journal *Stem Cells*, attributed this process to "accelerated repopulation," a term that refers to the increased growth rates of cancers during treatment gaps that far exceed their initial growth rates.[30]

In other words, cancer is significantly slower in its growth without the treatment that is supposed to eradicate it. Another study discusses the problem of tumor cell repopulation, recognized as a major challenge in treating cancers after radiation. This study suggested that dying cancer cells activate survival and proliferation signals, releasing growth factors to the surrounding living cancer cells.[31] Why Radiation only option?

Secondary Cancers from Chemotherapy and Radiation

Chemotherapy and radiation also increase the risk of developing secondary cancers. Although cancer survivors comprise about 3.5% of the population, subsequent malignancies among this group account for about 16% of all cancer incidence.[32] Secondary cancers are reported to be the sixth most common group of malignancies.[33] These can be recurrences of the original cancer type or a different type of cancer altogether.

Myelodysplastic syndrome (MDS) made U.S. headlines a few years ago when the news anchor Robin Roberts was diagnosed with this secondary cancer after treatment for breast cancer. MDS is a bone marrow disorder in which the bone marrow does not produce enough healthy blood cells. According to the MDS Foundation and the American Cancer Society, radiation and chemotherapy treatments for cancer are among the known triggers for the development of MDS. People who have received these treatments for cancers that are considered potentially curable, such as breast, testicular, Hodgkin's disease, and non-Hodgkin's lymphoma, are at risk of developing MDS for up to ten years following treatment. This secondary MDS often develops rapidly into acute leukemia.[34]

MDS is often treated with immunosuppressive therapy, chemotherapy, and bone marrow transplantation, further weakening the immune system and natural defenses against disease. In a report by Fox News Health, Elizabeth Griffiths, a physician at the Roswell Park Cancer Institute, speaking about MDS, said, "This disease is often the result of friendly fire accidentally sustained while a patient is being treated for another cancer."[35]

Chemotherapy and radiation may have their place in cancer treatment, but there is nothing "friendly" about them. There are many studies that have identified and discussed the risk of secondary cancers, especially in those people who have had relatively long-term survival after treatment for cancers that are considered potentially curable. Many of the studies that discuss secondary cancers include people who had both chemotherapy and radiation therapy, so it is difficult to know precisely which treatment contributed the most. The secondary cancers attributed to radiation therapy typically do not occur for many years, and it is understandable that people are willing to assume the risk of a second cancer in the future for a survival benefit in the present. It is, however, worth considering how large a survival benefit will be received and whether it is worth the future risk.

Although chemotherapy has demonstrated better success in treating the lymphoma known as Hodgkin's disease than it has with more common cancers, these survivors are known to be at substantially increased risk of secondary cancers. Young Hodgkin's survivors have an elevated risk of breast and colorectal cancer ten to twenty-five years before the age when routine screening would be recommended in the general population.[36]

A study in *The New England Journal of Medicine* reported that the incidence of a second cancer for these patients is 48.5% greater than those in the general population, even after forty years of surviving Hodgkin's lymphoma, and that these survivors also have an increased risk of cardiovascular disease.[37]

Second cancers are a leading cause of death among men who have been treated for testicular cancer, another cancer for which conventional oncology boasts high "cure" rates through the use of both chemotherapy and radiation. Testicular cancer survivors are at a significantly increased risk of solid tumors for at least thirty-five years after treatment. These cancers include those of the mesothelioma, esophagus, lung, colon, bladder, pancreas, and stomach.[38]

An article in the *Journal of the National Cancer Institute* reviewed previous studies to assess the risk of second cancers and cardiovascular disease following radiation therapy for a variety of cancers. Radiation therapy for cervical cancer was associated with significantly increased risk of cancers of the bladder, kidneys, rectum, uterus, and ovaries. The risk for several solid pelvic tumors was found to remain significantly elevated for more than forty years after radiation. The cancers associated with breast cancer radiation include those of the opposite breast, lung, and esophagus. The researchers found a higher incidence of secondary cancer in those who had a mastectomy, versus a lumpectomy, presumably due to the larger area of treatment. This study also identified that survivors of Hodgkin's lymphoma have the highest overall risk for secondary cancers. In a population of 2,742 survivors, 94% received radiation, and the thirty-year incidence of secondary cancers was 10.9% in males and 26.1% in females. Females had an 18.3% incidence of invasive breast cancer, with a median time of twenty-one years between treatment of Hodgkin's lymphoma and diagnosis of breast cancer.[39]

Radiation therapy for breast cancer is thought to decrease regional recurrence and improve overall survival, but unfortunately has been associated with an increased second cancer risk, sometimes decades after the radiation exposure. A 2016 review and analysis of twenty-two studies that comprised over half a million breast cancer patients was published in *Radiotherapy and Oncology*. It compared the cancer incidence of those who received radiation and those who did not, and for those who received radiation, the incidence of second cancers that included the lung, esophagus, thyroid, and connective tissues progressively increased over time, peaking at ten to fifteen years following diagnosis. The authors concluded that radiation for breast cancer is associated with an excess risk of a second non-breast cancer overall, and in organs adjacent to the previous treatment area.[40]

These articles and research findings are just a smattering of the evidence that exists about the risks and limited benefits of chemotherapy and radiation. There is no denying that these therapies can rapidly shrink tumors, and can be lifesaving when the tumor threatens essential organ function. Unfortunately, in most cases, reducing the size of a tumor does not translate into increased survival. It appears these treatments can instead contribute to metastasis and the progression of cancer, increase the risk of second cancers, weaken the immune system, and damage organs. For many people with late-stage cancers, chemo and radiation are ineffective, or only minimally effective, and, at best, increase survival by mere months. Understandably, they are used because the tumor-focused paradigm within which mainstream medicine operates has nothing better to offer. That is, possibly until now? Are newer cancer therapies indeed less risky and less toxic than chemotherapy and radiation?

Precision Medicine and Targeted Therapies

The image of a pile of big orange capsules referred to as "bullets" on the cover of *Time* magazine in 2001 was that of Gleevec, also known as imantinib, the first targeted therapy drug to be approved by the FDA. The discovery and use of Gleevec represented a quantum leap forward in the ability of physicians to treat chronic myelogenous leukemia, (CML) a relatively rare form of cancer. Before Gleevec, patients with CML were treated with chemotherapy and bone marrow transplants, and most survived for only two or three years. The use of Gleevec has resulted in a ten-year survival rate of 83%, and physicians and researchers are hopeful that most CML patients will now live out their full life spans. Unfortunately, targeted therapies for the most common malignancies have not had the success of Gleevec. Put simply, the genetic mutations found in CML are less complex and diverse than those found in other cancers. Despite the excitement in oncology at present due to the relatively new science of "precision medicine," it is still too soon to determine what overall contribution these new drug therapies will bring to cancer survival rates, as discussed in chapter 3.

Many of the targeted therapies are used in combination with each other, or with chemotherapy, and have side effects of their own. Although the side effects of targeted therapies are usually not quite as severe as those of chemotherapy, they are significant, the most common being diarrhea and liver problems such as hepatitis. Others include problems with blood clotting and wound healing, nausea and vomiting, high blood pressure, organ damage, second cancers, hair loss, fatigue, and increased risk of infections.[41]

Hormone Therapy

Hormone therapy is a type of targeted therapy used for those with prostate and breast cancer, cancers that rely upon sex hormones to grow. Drugs are used that block the body's ability to produce hormones or interfere with how hormones behave in the body, and are usually used in conjunction with other treatments. Although considered an important aspect of treatment for many women with breast cancer, the risks of hormone therapies are numerous, and some women are unable to continue treatment due to debilitating side effects. Many of these hormone therapies can cause blood clots, stroke, heart problems, joint pain, depression, and fatigue. Tamoxifen, one of the most widely used hormonal therapies, has been found to decrease the chance of estrogen-dependent breast cancer by 49%, but increase the risk of endometrial cancer by 150%.[42]

Immunotherapy

The immunotherapy drug Keytruda (pembrolizumab) made headlines in 2016 after former President Jimmy Carter was successfully treated with the drug for melanoma that had spread to his liver and brain. Keytruda was FDA approved in 2011 and is one of several immunotherapy drugs that act as a "checkpoint inhibitor," essentially preventing the immune system from turning off and allowing it to identify and fight any cancer in the body. Immunotherapies have had the most success so far in treating melanoma, but they are increasingly being used for other cancers, and there are hundreds of clinical trials studying the use of checkpoint inhibitors and other forms of immunotherapy.

Although the "checkpoint inhibitor" immunotherapy drugs have been miraculous in many cases, sometimes melting away tumors over short periods of time, there have been reports of death and severe, life-threatening side effects. Because these drugs essentially take the brakes off the immune system, the immune system can attack healthy organs, much as it does in auto-immune diseases. Oncologists at Yale University believe immunotherapy is causing a new type of acute-onset diabetes due to the effects of the checkpoint inhibitor drugs. Studies are finding that severe reactions occur nearly 20% of the time when one drug is used, and in more than 50% of patients when drugs are used in combination.[43]

Monoclonal antibodies are another type of immunotherapy used for some types of cancer. They are antibodies that bind to certain proteins or other substances on the surface of cancer cells, stimulating an immune response that can destroy cancer cells. They essentially serve as substitute antibodies that can restore, enhance, or mimic the immune system's attack on cancer cells. These drugs are made by a complex process that involves harvesting antibody-producing cells from mice and/or rats. Genetic engineering is used to replace as much rodent antibody as is possible with human antibody.[44]

In addition to the side effects common to many immunotherapies, such as flu-like symptoms and allergic reactions, many of these monoclonal antibody drugs can also cause secondary cancers, significant organ damage, and other serious problems. Some of these include cardiopulmonary arrest, bowel obstruction and perforation, kidney and liver toxicity, blood clots in the lungs, and infections, among others.[45]

The newest type of immunotherapy is called CAR-T, short for chimeric antigen receptor T-cell therapy. The first CAR-T therapy, Kymriah, received FDA approval in August 2017 for the treatment of those under age twenty-five with acute lymphoblastic leukemia who have not responded to standard treatment or who have suffered relapses. Yescarta, a CAR-T therapy approved for adults with certain types of large B-cell lymphoma who have not responded to other types of treatments, was FDA approved in October 2017. These treatments reprogram a patient's own immune cells to attack the cancer, and come with a hefty price tag. Kymriah costs $475,000 for the single required treatment, and Yescarta costs $373,000. Although there is much excitement about this new therapy, it is only available to adults with other cancers in clinical trials, and there have been reports of severe side effects and at least one death.[46]

How to Decide

Despite the known limitations and risks of conventional cancer treatment, making the decision to take another path is difficult for many people. Such a decision requires thorough research, as well as serious soul searching, a trust in one's own inner wisdom, and a hefty dose of courage. This decision may be easier for people like Valerie and Bailey, who ran out of options within conventional medicine, but taking the path less traveled can be frightening, despite the prognosis. Many people encounter strong resistance from friends and family who disagree with their decision to pursue a different course of treatment, even if it seems clear that conventional treatment will not result in improved survival. Reports in the media can create conflict and confusion, and doctors and the mainstream media talk about "evidence-based medicine" as if it were completely accurate and reliable, free from any sort of bias or corrupt science. Doctors may tell the patient that they are crazy for making an alternative choice, and have been known to say things like "If you don't do chemotherapy, you will die." The stories about how and why people chose another path despite such resistance and mixed messages are fascinating tales of chance encounters, spiritual experiences, and answers to prayers.

CHAPTER 5
Resistance, the Media, and "Evidence-Based" Medicine

Marie Halbrendt Carlson encountered very strong resistance to her decision to pursue alternative treatment when she was diagnosed with breast cancer. Her family and her doctors were against her choices, but Marie had a very influential chance encounter as well as a spiritual experience that guided her treatment decision. Marie is a wife, mother, and secretary at the police department in a small Massachusetts town. She is a soft-spoken woman with a relaxed demeanor, but is tenacious, stubborn, and tough as nails beneath the surface. Prior to Marie's experience with cancer, her friend Bonny had told her about a woman, Eva, who had been told by three doctors that amputating her cancer-ridden leg was the only way to save her life. Eva had flatly refused to lose her leg and instead went to a cancer clinic in Tijuana, despite her family's strong opposition to her choice. After hearing that Eva was now cancer-free and in possession of both legs after her trip to Mexico, Marie decided that should she ever be diagnosed with cancer, she would go to the same Tijuana clinic for treatment.

A few years later, Marie had a routine mammogram, only because her new doctor insisted upon it. A lump was found, and a lumpectomy with biopsy was scheduled. Although Marie tried to convince herself that the lump was nothing, thoughts about the possibility of cancer never left her. She thought back to the story she had been told about Eva and arranged a phone call with her before the lumpectomy. Marie was amazed to discover that twenty years had passed since Eva had received treatment at the Tijuana clinic, and that she continued to be healthy and cancer-free. The next day Marie called the clinic and spoke with one of the doctors. She decided then that this clinic, the Bio-Medical Center, was where she would go, should the lump be malignant.

Marie discussed this plan with her daughter, Marta, an outgoing and energetic married mother of two young children. Marta did not believe that her mother's lump would prove to be cancerous, so she readily promised Marie that were it cancer, she would accompany her to Mexico. After Marie received the news that, yes, it was breast cancer, Marie describes feeling very calm and almost transcendent—that she was somehow guided to make the decision to take an alternative treatment path. When Marta was told about her mother's cancer, she honored her promise, despite having strong reservations about the decision. When Marie told her typically kind and supportive husband of her plans, he was horrified. Both he and Marie's son ardently tried to convince her that she was making a huge mistake by not following the recommendations of her doctors. It was a subject of tireless dissension and argument in the household, but Marie stayed firm with the decision that felt right in her whole being. Two weeks later, much to her husband's chagrin, she left for Mexico with her daughter.

In contrast to Marie's reserved and quiet nature, Marta is the kind of person who can and will strike up a conversation with anyone, anywhere. While Marie was being evaluated at the Bio-Medical Center in Tijuana, Marta spoke with many of the other patients and heard numerous success stories about the Hoxsey treatment that is offered exclusively at the Bio-Medical Center. Marta became convinced of the wisdom of her mother's decision, and accompanied her on follow-up visits.

I spoke with Marie's husband recently, and based on that conversation, it is hard to believe that he had given Marie such grief about her decision. He is now an ardent supporter of A/I approaches to cancer treatment, and he is fully aware of the problems with the cancer industry in the United States. Marie has been cancer-free for at least twelve years now, and is an advocate for the Bio-Medical Center. Marie authored *Yes You Can Say No*, a book about her experience with cancer, her physicians, and treatment at the Bio-Medical center.

Alternative vs. Conventional Polarity

Unlike Marie, who did not tell any of her friends or co-workers about her choice and felt so secure in her decision that she did not seek other opinions, many other people are subject to vast amounts of conflicting information and points of view. In addition to receiving input from various doctors, family members, and friends, most people who research cancer treatment options turn to the internet. A Google search for "alternative therapy for cancer" produces millions of results, with a mix of advertisements, government websites, and various articles which are either pro or anti alternative medicine.

Those who do research alternatives to standard methods of treating cancer will notice a somewhat uncivil dialogue between the proponents of nontoxic "alternative" or integrative treatment and conventional medical treatment. There seems to be no other disease that creates such a sharp divide between two dramatically different and, at times, dogmatic ideologies. The "alternative" side accuses standard medicine of being mercenary in their pursuit of profit in service of personal and corporate interests, and the conventional side accuses "alternative" medicine of selling unproven fraudulent cancer cures to desperate, gullible, and fearful cancer patients.

Even well-credentialed physicians and other practitioners of integrative and alternative medicine are often referred to as quacks, a word taken from the Dutch *kwakzalver*, meaning a hawker of salves. A quack is more commonly defined in dictionaries as "a fraudulent or ignorant pretender to medical skill" or "a person who pretends to have skills, knowledge or qualifications that he or she does not possess." According to this definition, well-trained and educated physicians are unfairly and inaccurately called "quacks," simply because they have used their knowledge in a manner that challenges dominant medical opinion and dogma.

Both the conventional and alternative sides sensationalize tidbits of information, which rarely tell the whole story. It can be very difficult to know who to believe, and to make decisions grounded in knowledge and common sense. In the midst of the debate, there are brilliant and dedicated integrative physicians, including some oncologists, all of whom originally came from the same type of medical training as their more conventionally oriented peers. I know from experience that it is all too easy to end up feeling conflicted and confused, as the writings of both camps are quite convincing. People with cancer just want to know the truth—they want to know what treatment gives them the best chance of success and a high quality of life, with minimal disability and risk from the treatments.

The Quack-Calling Media

Sciencebasedmedicine.org is a large and active website dedicated to discrediting non-standard approaches to treating disease, including cancer. The editors of this website, physicians Steven Novella and David Gorski, along with other physicians, make antagonistic attacks on the most benign therapies. Their attacks bring to mind the story of Ignaz Semmelweis, a Hungarian obstetrician practicing in Vienna in the 1800s. He was attacked and ridiculed by his peers for suggesting that doctors should wash their hands before delivering a baby. Semmelweis accurately believed that the doctors carried some sort of morbid poison on their hands after performing autopsies, since the deliveries assisted by midwives did not result in the same high maternal death rate from puerperal fever. He was advocating his discovery well before the medical profession was ready to accept it, and before the technology existed to prove it.

Gorski criticizes the movement of many of his peers toward integrative oncology, he attacks the scientists who release data and publish papers critical of genetically modified foods, and he criticizes the large well-known cancer centers that have established CAM (complementary and alternative medicine) or integrative medicine programs. He calls fellow physicians "quacks" or "uber-quacks" if they don't think or practice like he does. Novella also voices his concern about the large cancer centers that increasingly offer complementary and integrative medicine programs, and says, "We've become witch doctors."[1]

Evidence-Based Medicine?

Authors and doctors such as Gorski and Novella reject anything that does not have the benefit of a clinical trial to back it up, but even commonly used and accepted medical treatments in use today are not all supported by sufficient reliable evidence. An analysis in *The British Medical Journal* identified that 47% of commonly accepted medical treatments are unknown in their effectiveness, and 10% were identified as being likely to be harmful or unlikely to be beneficial.[2] In an article providing commentary on these findings, author Dana Ullman points out that whatever has been in vogue in conventional medicine in one decade has often been declared ineffective, dangerous, and sometimes barbaric in later times, yet "alternatives" to this ever-changing treatment are called quackery, whether or not the defenders of "scientific medicine" know anything at all about these "alternative" treatments.[3]

An article in *The New York Times* titled "Believing in Treatments that Don't Work"[4] described several medical practices that continue despite evidence that they don't work or are harmful. According to the author, physician David H. Newman, "the practice of medicine contains countless examples of elegant medical theories that belie the best available evidence." Newman provides the example of early administration of beta-blockers to heart attack victims. This practice is not supported by evidence, yet because in theory it made sense, it continued to be done for years as a part of standard protocol. Although cough syrups are routinely advised by physicians, no cough remedies have ever been proven better than a placebo, either for adults or children. The use of stem-cell transplantation in women with high-risk breast cancer was an example of a cancer treatment that did not prove to be effective and was discontinued. High-dose chemotherapy and stem cell transplantation became a common, costly, and controversial practice for more than a decade, yet no improvement in survival was found.[5] Only four clinical trials were done, and three of them found the procedure did not improve survival. In his book *How We Do Harm: A Doctor Breaks Ranks About Being Sick in America*, oncologist Otis Brawley says that at least twenty-three thousand women underwent high-dose chemo with stem cell transplantation between 1989 and 2001, despite the fact that only a very small number of

American women had participated in a clinical trial of this procedure. Brawley writes that Werner Bezwoda, lead investigator of the only study that found favorable survival rates, became a pioneer of the procedure. It was later discovered that Bezwoda had created a completely fraudulent randomized clinical trial. This one study resulted in physicians around the world citing his results and charging insurers for the highly toxic "Bezwoda Regimen."[6]

As there are so many reports about how corrupt the whole business of clinical trials is, to call the results of these trials "evidence-based" can be completely misguided. A large majority of drug clinical trials are funded by pharmaceutical companies that are free to withhold the results of the trials that do not show their product to have a beneficial effect, yet publish the trials that do show a positive effect.[7] In addition, author Clifton Leaf, in his book *The Truth in Small Doses: Why We're Losing the War on Cancer and How to Win It*, reports that patients are selected for clinical trials based on who is most likely to have a favorable response and less likely to have an adverse event. This practice prevents many of the patients for whom the drug is designed from participating in the clinical trial. Leaf also reports that clinical trial recruitment strategies use inclusion criteria that are so selective that the possibility of adverse effects being seen are "engineered out."[8] Alarmingly, Leaf states that drug companies pay doctors for each patient they bring to a clinical trial, a seemingly huge conflict of interest.

Cancer drugs are often approved by the FDA with scanty evidence of their effectiveness, despite the huge price tags attached to them. Avastin was the first approved drug to interfere with the process of how tumors form and maintain a blood supply (angiogenesis). It was approved in 2004 after it showed that it extended patient survival in colon cancer by an average of 4.6 months. It received accelerated approval to be used in women with metastatic breast cancer, earning the drug company about a billion dollars in annual sales, despite the fact that there was no evidence that it worked for women with metastatic breast cancer.[9] Avastin, which costs about $100,000 per year, has become one of the most popular drugs in the world, with sales of about $3.5 billion a year, despite the fact that it may add only months, not years, to survival.[10]

The unfortunate reality is that a large clinical trial will never be undertaken on a treatment, or treatment program, that does not have the potential to greatly profit a corporate interest. Several of the doctors I spoke with in Mexico were confident that were a clinical trial to be conducted on a comprehensive A/I approach, the results would be far better than any of the drugs being trialed, including the new targeted and immunotherapy drugs that have received so much media attention. Such clinical trials will likely never be done in the United States due to the expense and lack of big-money interests required to fund them.

Media Bias and Big Pharma

The major media outlets are also biased against non-standard approaches to cancer treatment, as they are dependent on the pharmaceutical companies for much of their profit in the form of advertising. The website www.drugwatch.com, and numerous other sources, report that pharmaceutical companies spend more on marketing than they do on research and development, with billions of dollars spent on advertising that benefits the major print and television media companies. Research has shown that spending for ads for pharmaceutical products on television has grown 62% since 2012. One analysis showed that 72% of commercial breaks on the CBS Evening News program contain at least one pharmaceutical advertisement.[11]

The pharmaceutical companies also spend a hefty percentage of their billions of marketing dollars in the form of gifts and perks to a majority of U.S. physicians, hoping to influence their prescribing preferences. Although drug companies spent more than $3 billion a year marketing to consumers in the U.S. in 2012, this number is dwarfed by the estimated $24 billion they spent marketing to health care professionals.[12] Pfizer, one of the world's largest drug makers, paid about $20 million to 4,500 doctors and other medical professionals for consulting and speaking on the company's behalf in just the last six months of 2009, which was its first public disclosure of payments to the professionals who decide which drugs to recommend to patients. This disclosure did not include payments disbursed outside the United States.[13]

An interesting, or should I say irrational, study was published in August 2017 in the *Journal of the National Cancer Institute* titled "Use of Alternative Medicine for Cancer and Its Impact on Survival."[14] Popular media outlets quickly jumped on this study, including CNN, whose headline read "Choosing Alternative Cancer Therapy Doubles Risk of Death, Study Says."[15] The researchers, most of whom have received funding from pharmaceutical companies, selected 280 patients diagnosed between 2004 and 2013 who had chosen alternative medicine, and compared their survival rates with 560 patients who had received conventional cancer treatment for breast, prostate, lung, and colorectal cancer. The researchers did not define alternative medicine, a broad and murky term that could include any number of therapies such as crystals, vitamins, or consuming only wheat grass juice. In addition, the study criteria for inclusion were patients who used unproven cancer treatments administered by non-medical personnel. Since all of the therapies offered by reputable alternative and integrative doctors and clinics are administered by medical personnel, it is hard to fathom how such a study has any relevance to those who receive care from licensed and qualified professionals.

The headline to this story could easily (and more accurately) have been "Conventional Cancer Treatment Is No More Effective Than Alternative Therapy for Prostate Cancer," as the difference in survival of prostate cancer patients who used unknown alternative therapies was statistically insignificant. The patients who used "alternative" medicine for all four cancer types studied also had a more advanced stage of cancer than those in the group who had only conventional treatment, making a comparison even less relevant. Researchers were confounded by the fact that patients in the alternative medicine group were more likely to be female, and have a higher income and educational level than those who chose only conventional treatment.

To provide expert commentary on this study, CNN chose the most biased and anti-alternative medicine physician they could find, quack-caller David Gorski, of sciencebasedmedicine.org. Popular natural health blogger and cancer survivor Chris Wark provided commentary on this study on his website, calling it a "straw man study," pointing out its many weaknesses as well as revealing the depth of the conflicts of interest of the involved researchers.[16]

The Alternative Cancer Treatment Media

The alternative cancer treatment media can also distort or exaggerate facts to convince us of the wisdom of their platform. A common and well-circulated recent example is the headline that exclaims "Seventy-Five Percent of Oncologists Would Not Accept Chemotherapy for Themselves or Their Families." Few of the authors of the subsequent "anti-chemo" articles mention the details of this small survey that was administered to oncologists during a conference at McGill University in 1985. The survey asked the attendees whether they would accept Cisplatin for non-small-cell lung cancer. Cisplatin had not been trialed on this type of cancer; hence there was no evidence that it would be effective. A follow-up survey was done twelve years later, in 1997, and the proportion of oncologists that would accept chemotherapy was far higher. I don't doubt that there are oncologists who would not accept chemotherapy, but there are no published contemporary surveys proving that a majority would refuse it. There was a more recent study published indicating that if terminally ill, most physicians would refuse the high-intensity medical interventions they administer to their terminally ill patients.[17] This study did not specifically name chemotherapy as one of the interventions, however. I am not a fan of chemotherapy, and have already stated that I would not accept it, but these deceptive headlines and articles based on studies at least twenty years old fuel the quack-callers' arguments about how deceptive and misguided the proponents of alternative cancer treatment can be in an alleged attempt to rob the sick, dying, and desperate of their money.

Yet another widely circulated research finding in the alternative cancer treatment media is one featuring the headline "Study Finds That Untreated Cancer Patients Live Four Times Longer than Those Who Are Treated" and refers to the research of scientist Hardin Jones, whose data collection revealed that people with cancer who refused conventional treatment lived longer than those who submitted to conventional treatment. The research of Jones was impressive, and is food for thought and further research, but this research was presented to the American Cancer Society's Annual Science Writers Conference in 1969, and Jones's research spanned approximately the twenty years prior to 1969. Again, this reliance on outdated research only strengthens attempts by quack-callers to portray how desperate proponents of alternative medicine are, resorting to presenting such old research as currently relevant information. One could argue that cancer treatment has changed little in the past fifty years, especially for later-stage disease, and people do continue to die from conventional treatments rather than the cancer itself. In fact, the report of a 2016 study concluded that Stage II colon cancer patients who received chemotherapy were more likely to have poor quality of life, recurrence, and all-cause mortality after twenty-four months compared to those who did not receive chemotherapy.[18]

Physicians today are demonstrably better at keeping patients alive while they attempt to kill the cancer than they were fifty years ago, if only because lifesaving technologies have been developed in the past five decades that have had an impact on survival, such as powerful antibiotics and more sophisticated monitoring equipment and diagnostics, among other refinements of medical practice in general. Even though many of the chemotherapy drugs in use today were used fifty years ago, their administration is more carefully prescribed and monitored. It was thirty-six years ago that I administered Cisplatin and other chemotherapy drugs without the benefit of intravenous infusion pumps. I cannot help but wonder how many patients I may have inadvertently infused with these toxic drugs too rapidly because I became too busy with other patients to check the infusion as often as I should have. Over the past fifty years, vast improvements in surgical techniques and refinements in radiation therapy have also contributed to keeping the patient alive longer for the benefit of everyone, including those who get their paycheck through employment in the cancer industry.

Self-Treatment as a Possible Alternative to Conventional Treatment

I support the movement toward seeking professional alternative and integrative cancer treatment, especially for those whose treatment would consist primarily of chemotherapy, but I have concerns about the polarity this revolution is creating. Many more people are attempting to treat their own cancer based on information they find in books and online, reading the "miracle" testimonies of other patients who treated their own cancer naturally. I do not agree with the quack-caller inferences that people diagnosed with cancer are desperate, gullible, and not capable of rational judgment, but I know there are many people who cannot afford A/I treatment or do not have access to a qualified practitioner to monitor and guide them while still rejecting most or all conventional treatment.

I recently consulted with a few people who were adamantly against chemotherapy and radiation and were attempting to treat and even diagnose their own cancer. One woman, Jane, had an aggressive form of uterine cancer. From the information Jane read on various natural health websites, including testimonies of people who had been "cured" using home therapies, she had been attempting to treat her own cancer. She had read of many people who had achieved remission with diet alone and had attempted to do the same. She was taking a few supplements that she had heard were helpful in treating cancer and she was alkalinizing her water. I spoke with Jane shortly after she had had extensive surgery to remove the tumor invading her bladder and ureters, which had made urination impossible. She most definitely wanted to live, despite the recommendations of her surgeon that she consider hospice if she was not willing to be treated with chemotherapy. I assumed she wanted to speak with me to learn about professional A/I treatment options, but I soon realized she was hoping I had suggestions for additional "DIY" (do it yourself) therapies that she could incorporate. As gently as I could, I urged Jane to pursue professional treatment of any kind to keep her alive. She alluded to an unhappy marriage and not having the funds and freedom to travel to an integrative clinic. I recommended a well-known integrative physician located an hour away from where she lived, who had years of experience treating cancer. I offered to provide recovery consult sessions gratis to help Jane create a healing plan that addressed the non-medical aspects of recovering from cancer. I never heard back from her. It was a very sad situation.

Could it be that conventional treatment for an aggressive and fast-growing cancer is better than inadequate or no treatment? Would it be feasible to undergo conventional treatment for a cancer such as Jane's, and later do A/I treatment to recover from the ill effects of conventional treatment, improve overall health, and decrease the likelihood of a recurrence? During one trip to Tijuana, I met Hope, who was doing just that.

When I met her in Tijuana, Hope appeared to be a strong and healthy woman in her forties. In fact, the only clue that she might be ill was the very fine hair that she wore shortly cropped, which led me to believe she had lost her hair from chemotherapy at some point in the not too distant past. Hope had just completed A/I treatment and was going home the following day. During a phone call a few months later, I learned that Hope is a very successful woman, the CEO of a small Boston company that she built from the ground up. Hope had been diagnosed with Stage IV endometrial cancer about eight months before I met her. She had had breast cancer ten years prior, and had been taking Tamoxifen, which carries a small risk of uterine cancer for the women who take it. The information given to Hope about Tamoxifen warned of the risk, but said that any developing endometrial cancer is discovered very early. Hope faithfully went for the recommended six-month checkups since starting Tamoxifen, and was dismayed that her doctor did not discover the endometrial cancer until it had metastasized to Stage IV disease. Hope went through surgery, chemotherapy, and radiation for this new cancer, but knew that even though she had been told there was no detectable cancer following the treatment, her chances of long-term survival were poor, and recurrence was a clear possibility.

Many of the stories of people I have met on their journey through cancer contain an interesting twist—a chance meeting or event that determines their next step—and Hope's was no exception. Around the time of the uterine cancer diagnosis, Hope's brother-in-law went to an industry conference and just happened to meet Bailey O'Brien (see chapter 1), who told him of her successful treatment in Mexico and offered to speak with Hope. Hope contacted Bailey to discuss the treatment Bailey had received, and after doing further research, made the decision to go to Tijuana after undergoing conventional treatment at home.

As I spoke with Hope, I was surprised to discover that when I had met her in Tijuana, where she appeared well-nourished and healthy, she had completed chemotherapy only about a month prior. Hope described many of the things she did while undergoing treatment that helped her to avoid the worst of the side effects during chemotherapy and radiation, including coffee enemas and various supplements. Hope was continuing to administer two of the immunotherapies used at the clinic in Tijuana and was following a modified Gerson diet. All the juicing of vegetables was proving very time consuming, and although she felt healthy and was back to working full-time, Hope expressed that the fear of a cancer recurrence continued to be an unwelcome presence in her life.

Hope had mixed feelings about the time she spent in Mexico, receiving treatment. Her doctor wanted her to return for three days every month for a full year to continue treatments, but the cost and time away from work and family was unacceptable. She returned home feeling lost and very much on her own to manage her health. Her oncologist did not approve of the therapies from Mexico that she was taking, and he wanted her to begin Avastin, a drug that has numerous side effects and is frequently prescribed to slow the growth of the blood vessels that feed cancer. After Hope's experience with Tamoxifen, she wanted nothing to do with another drug that could just make things worse. She finally found an experienced integrative oncology physician located about ninety minutes from her home, and was going to his clinic twice weekly for intravenous vitamin C and other therapies to strengthen her immune system and help prevent recurrence. Hope felt relieved that she now had a local physician to monitor her and help her efforts to stay healthy.

Making the Decision

In her book, *Radical Remission: Surviving Cancer Against All Odds*, psychologist Kelly A. Turner identified nine key factors that were common among the thousands of people she studied who defied a terminal diagnosis with a complete reversal of their disease. One of these key factors was "Taking Control of Your Health," and Turner found that this included taking an active role, being willing to make life changes, and being able to cope with resistance.[19] Another key factor was "Following Your Intuition." Both of these are essential when making the decision whether to passively follow conventional medical advice, choose alternative therapies, or combine both approaches.

Part of taking an active role is being willing to do the research, being comfortable asking many questions of a doctor, and being prepared to find another doctor if he or she is not willing to take the time necessary to engage the patient as a partner in treatment. Obviously, choosing a support person who can help with these tasks can be invaluable. Many patients say they felt rushed into treatment by oncologists and their staff, despite the fact that, for most people, the urgency is unwarranted. Unless the tumor is in a location that presents an imminent threat to life or essential bodily functions, there is time to carefully weigh all the options.

There are many questions that should be asked of an oncologist that are essential to making a decision about treatment choice. Aside from the basics, such as knowing the exact diagnosis, stage, prognosis, and proposed treatment, other questions can be more revealing of the oncologist's overall method of working with a patient. The most important question to ask could be: *Is this proposed treatment curative or palliative?* As mentioned in chapter 4, many oncologists will recommend aggressive chemotherapy, despite knowing the chances of long-term remission for a particular type and stage of cancer are extremely poor. It is important to know whether the oncologist is open to, and supportive of, those who consider using integrative and alternative therapies, and whether he or she is willing to treat them if these are used. For those who are considering alternative therapies and/or lifestyle changes exclusively, it is essential to ask whether the doctor is willing to provide monitoring and diagnostic testing if a patient initially declines the recommended treatment. The answers to these questions can be real deal-breakers, and will reveal the doctor's general attitudes toward therapies that support the health of the person with cancer, rather than exclusively focusing on shrinking tumors at any cost.

Another aspect of "Taking Control of Your Health" is being willing to honestly evaluate one's lifestyle, and deciding how much change is possible and desirable. Choosing an alternative path in cancer treatment requires far more personal responsibility and commitment, whether that involves changing dietary patterns, reducing stress, letting go of toxic relationships and situations, and/or deepening social and spiritual connection. People with cancer are often subject to the opinions of many other people, including friends, family, and health care professionals. Having strong personal boundaries and being able to remain firm in a commitment to the chosen recovery and healing plan is optimal for those who choose to forge their own path. For those whose boundaries are not as strong, and who have difficulty standing firm against the resistance of others, a more formal A/I treatment program directed by a trusted physician might be a better choice to consider, especially if financially and geographically viable.

Being able to access and follow one's intuition regarding treatment choice has been described as essential by many people who have recovered from cancer. This requires devoting time to get out of the state of mental analysis that is necessary when researching treatment options and making the time to tune into gut feelings that are informed by self-awareness, insight, and knowledge. It is beyond the scope of this book to describe the many ways people can learn to access their "sixth sense," and it often differs from individual to individual. Learning to quiet the mind through prayer, meditation, conscious breathing, and walks in nature can be a place to start.

Those who are interested in a holistic approach to treating cancer, and are prepared to take control of their treatment, often start with an evaluation of how their diet may have contributed to their illness. Fundamental to all A/I cancer treatment, whether in the United States or abroad, is an emphasis on nutrition and its role in recovery. Without a commitment to adopting an anti-cancer diet, the success of other therapies, whether conventional, integrative, or alternative, are likely to be short-lived. Physicians receive little to no education about nutrition in their formal training, and conventional oncologists often tell patients to eat whatever they want, ignoring or being unaware of the volumes of nutritional research pertinent to cancer. There is also debate about what dietary strategy is most effective for recovery from cancer, with equally qualified professionals recommending one approach over another. This debate can often seem like a microcosm of the polarity that exists between conventional and alternative cancer treatment, and some of the same decision-making strategies will apply.

CHAPTER 6
Nutritional and Metabolic Approaches to Cancer

There is an invisible dynamic civilization going about its daily life within you right now. The approximately 100 trillion members of this civilization represent up to two thousand species of living organisms that have lived and evolved with humans for millions of years. The cells of these busy ecosystems make up 90% of the cells in your body, and if packaged, would be about the size of your brain. Their colonies create separate ecosystems, which at this moment are sending instructions throughout your body, influencing your physical and mental health. This civilization, made up of bacteria, viruses, and other microorganisms, is collectively known as the microbiota, or microbiome. The microbiome is a control center for many aspects of our biology, and plays an important role in immune function, digestion, metabolism, and emotional stability. The microbiome is estimated to possess a thousand more genes than its human host, and although this is a very new science, researchers believe that the microbiome has an effect on human genes due to epigenetics.

Epigenetics is the name of the new science that explores the effect of the environment on cellular behavior and how our genes behave, referred to as "gene expression." Gene expression is the process by which proteins are manufactured from instructions stored in the DNA, which can make certain genes active or inactive. By making changes in some aspect of our environment, we now know that we can change how our genes are expressed. An even newer research field is the science of nutrigenomics. Nutrigenomics investigates how nutrients affect gene and protein expression and influence cellular metabolism, and intersects with the study of the microbiome.

Studies of the composition of the microbiome of people who live in societies where there is far less cancer, heart disease, and other chronic illness have found a greater diversity and different composition of organisms compared to those who live in industrialized society. Scientists are just beginning to study the relationship between cancer and a varied and healthy microbiome. They have found the strongest connection between colon cancer and characteristics of the microbiome, but studies involving other cancers have also suggested a relationship.[1]

What creates the most robust and diverse microbiome? It is no surprise that scientists have found that those who consume a high-fiber, plant-based diet have the most varied and abundant microbiome. Those who have taken frequent doses of antibiotics, or who consume animals that have been fed antibiotics (as is common in the U.S. commercial meat industry), have a less diverse microbiome. Justin Sonnenburg, a microbiologist at Stanford and a leading researcher of the microbiome and its relationship to health and disease, believes that diet and the resulting microbiome of modern western civilization predisposes individuals to a variety of diseases. He suggests that interactions between microbes and human hosts may explain several diseases that share inflammation as a common basis, including cancer.[2]

Although still a newer research interest, the study of the microbiome is beginning to accumulate data that can inform dietary choices for any chronic disease. In the future, nutrigenomics may be able to tell us precisely what foods turn certain cancer genes on or off. For now, there is plenty of research about the properties of certain foods and how they affect cancer cells, which will be discussed later in this chapter. When considering the various nutritional approaches used to prevent or treat cancer, the question of how a particular diet will affect the microbiome is relevant in light of the research done to date.

Within the world of alternative and integrative treatment for cancer, there is considerable debate about what represents the best diet to prevent and target cancer. Many nutritional plans have been recommended, including the paleo diet, the Weston Price diet, metabolic typing diets, the macrobiotic diet, the Budwig diet, and diets based on blood type. These may all have some merit, but it is the ketogenic diet, the Mediterranean diet, Gerson Therapy, the plant-based diet, and raw vegan diet that appear to have garnered the most attention in the media and among doctors and patients.

The Ketogenic Diet

In recent years, the ketogenic diet has received enormous attention by cancer researchers, A/I (alternative/integrative) practitioners, and health-focused authors. Although none of the A/I doctors in Tijuana that I spoke with said they recommended the ketogenic diet, some of the patients that I met in Mexico were following it, and several American A/I physicians who are known for treating cancer recommend it. The internet offers countless articles, videos, and books touting the benefits of the ketogenic diet for cancer, as well as for weight loss and chronic degenerative diseases. The ketogenic diet has received a lot of attention for its use in cancer treatment due to the work of biologist Thomas Seyfried, a professor at Boston College and author of *Cancer as a Metabolic Disease: On the Origin, Management, and Prevention of Cancer*. Seyfried has also written many papers and given many interviews and presentations about the metabolic cause of cancer and how the ketogenic diet targets cancer.[3]

Cancer cells are known to be "obligate glucose metabolizers," often using far more glucose to produce energy than normal cells. Recall the theories of Otto Warburg, the German physician and Nobel laureate, who identified that cancer cells thrive in an environment of low oxygen, using fermentation rather than respiration to create energy. Fermentation is a primitive process that uses glucose but does not require oxygen. The mitochondria in cancer cells is damaged, preventing cancer cells from using oxygen to produce energy as normal cells do. Restriction of carbohydrates, which break down into glucose, is thought to create severe stress to cancer cells. Normal cells can adapt to the deprivation of glucose, using ketone bodies for their energy. Ketone bodies are byproducts created by the liver as a result of the body using fat for energy.

Since cancer cells are known to use more glucose than normal cells, the carbohydrates that break down into glucose are severely restricted in the ketogenic diet. Protein must also be restricted on the ketogenic diet, as excessive protein creates an abundance of the amino acid glutamine, which is known to fuel cancer growth. Protein can also be used by the liver to create glucose, and excessive protein can also activate a biological pathway called mTor, known to contribute to the development of many cancers. The goal in the ketogenic diet is to have a consistent blood glucose level of 55–70 mgdl (milligrams per deciliter), and a ketone level of two to five milimolar, measured by the relatively inexpensive home glucose and ketone meters that diabetics often use to measure their blood sugar and determine the amount of insulin they need.

The ketogenic diet is 75–85% fat, 10–20% protein, and only about 5% carbohydrate. For cancer patients, this very low carbohydrate count is coupled with total calorie restriction. For a middle-aged woman of average size and activity level, this would translate into a total daily carbohydrate intake of about 15 grams, or 60 calories coming from carbohydrate. This is a very extreme restriction, and represents the amount of carbs that would be found in about two-and-one-half cups of chopped broccoli, or half of a small potato. Some physician authors recommend only restricting "net carbs" rather than total carbs. The "net" carbohydrate count refers to the total grams of carbs minus the grams of fiber, as fiber content does not raise blood sugar. Even using this formula, the diet is highly restrictive—that half of a small potato still contains about 12 grams of carbs after the amount of fiber is subtracted. On the ketogenic diet, high-quality saturated fats such as coconut oil, avocados, and organic butter are preferred due to their ability to create a higher level of ketone bodies as compared to unsaturated fats such as olive oil.

What is often not mentioned in the media that recommend the ketogenic diet for cancer is the need for total calorie restriction. Seyfried states that it is the reduction of one's total daily calories by about 40% that creates the benefits of the ketogenic diet for cancer. Seyfried views the ketogenic diet as a therapeutic fast that can be maintained safely by most people over an extended period of time. He has also mentioned in one of his many lectures that a raw vegan diet can result in the body using ketones for fuel and have the same anti-cancer effect, but that because fat is satiating, it "takes the sting out of a therapeutic fast."[4]

This therapeutic fast is reported to have profound effects on reducing and weakening cancer cells, and mimics the metabolic physiology of starvation without actually causing starvation. The therapeutic fast is reported to prevent or slow down the process of angiogenesis, whereby tumors create their blood supply. It is reported to cause apoptosis, meaning that cancer cells die off, and it is anti-inflammatory. Seyfried says that a high-fat, moderate-protein, ultra-low-carbohydrate diet that provides adequate calories will not have the same effect as that of a proportionally identical yet calorie-restricted diet on blood glucose levels and the production of ketone bodies, essential for the cancer-weakening effect. He explains that the amount of fat that would be consumed adhering to an adequate-calorie ketogenic diet would be excessive, and since excessive fats can be made into glycerol, a form of glucose, the calorie restriction is essential to keep blood sugar low and ketones high.

Seyfried feels strongly that those who choose to go on the ketogenic diet should be under the care of a health professional who understands the process and is able to monitor its effects. He says that individuals can have issues with electrolyte changes and side effects, and that some should not even attempt the diet. He reports that some people should embark on the ketogenic diet in phases, while being medically monitored as the diet is fine-tuned. Many people have withdrawal symptoms from the effects of low glucose in the brain, similar to withdrawing from drugs, as the brain breaks its addiction to glucose. Seyfried admits that the ketogenic diet is very difficult for the majority of people, and that there are not enough knowledgeable health care practitioners available to monitor those who attempt the diet for the control of cancer. He says that the diet is simple in concept, but much more difficult to implement. Although Seyfried is vocal about his lack of confidence in all the investments in researching targeted therapies for the multitudes of genetic mutations found in cancer cells, he is not at all against using drugs. He feels that more research should be directed toward drugs and treatments that target the mitochondrial dysfunction common to all cancer cells. He sees the ketogenic diet as a strategy to slow down the growth of the tumor and make it vulnerable to lower, less toxic doses of available drugs.[5]

So, is there any science that points to the effectiveness of the ketogenic diet for cancer beyond its theoretical underpinnings? There have not been any large human clinical trials of the ketogenic diet for cancer, likely due to a lack of research funding versus a lack of interest among scientists. The sparse amount of research that has been done has focused on glioblastoma multiforme, an aggressive and usually fatal brain cancer. There are a few case studies in the medical literature that point to the benefit of the restricted-calorie ketogenic diet for humans with cancer, and these studies also underline the difficulty of compliance with the diet. A German study evaluated a calorie-restricted ketogenic diet in sixteen patients with end-stage malignant tumors of various types who had exhausted all standard cancer therapies. Only five of the sixteen were able to complete three months of treatment due to difficulty with compliance, and all five had positive outcomes, with no tumor progression while on the diet.[6] To my knowledge there was no follow-up of these five patients to determine the degree of tumor progression, if and when they discontinued the diet.

A single case report exists of a sixty-five-year-old woman with glioblastoma multiforme who had already received standard therapies and had significant tumor shrinkage after two months on the diet, to the point where the tumor could no longer be seen on MRI or PET scans. Ten weeks after the calorie-restricted keto diet was terminated, the tumor returned and the patient died shortly afterward.[7] There have also been mice studies that have shown the benefit of a ketogenic diet on reducing cancer progression and improving survival. A study that combined a ketogenic diet with supplemental ketones and hyperbaric oxygen showed that the mice receiving the combination therapy had a marked reduction in tumor growth rate and metastatic spread, and lived twice as long as the control group of mice.[8]

Seyfried, as well as some A/I physicians and other scientists, sees great potential for treating cancer by combining the calorie-restricted ketogenic diet with nontoxic therapies and lower doses of drugs. There has been research that suggests that fasting before and after receiving conventional cancer treatment enhances the treatment's effects and decreases toxicity to healthy cells.[9] It is also accepted in the scientific community that calorie restriction has the potential to prevent cancer and increase survival in cancer patients.[10]

Leigh Erin Connealy is an experienced integrative physician who is the director of the Cancer Center for Healing, in California, and author of the book *The Cancer Revolution*. Dr. Connealy expresses enthusiasm for the ketogenic diet for people with cancer, but she also acknowledges that some patients do better on a more moderate whole-foods plant-based diet with an increased but not excessive amount of carbohydrates. In her book she speaks to the fact that different people have different metabolisms, and while some people are able to avoid blood sugar spikes with 30–40 grams of carbohydrates a day, others have to limit daily carb intake to only 10 grams.[11] A blood sugar spike would indicate that the person is not using ketones for fuel.

Despite the fact that there are many researchers and doctors who are extremely enthusiastic about the role the ketogenic diet may play in healing cancer, many other doctors and scientists have concerns and reservations about the wisdom and validity of this approach. Physician and author John McDougall has been a loud voice for the benefits of a high-carbohydrate, low-fat diet, free of animal products, for over forty years. He is joined in his views by other senior nutritional medicine physicians and researchers, such as Neil Barnard, Dean Ornish, Caldwell Esselstyn, T. Colin Campbell, and Michael Greger. McDougall is concerned about the recent promotion of low-carbohydrate diets to prevent and treat cancer, and states "these diets consist of the very foods known to cause cancers of the breast, colon, and prostate."[12] He acknowledges that it is widely accepted in the scientific community that inducing a metabolic state of starvation by restricting total calories, regardless of whether they derive from fat, carbs, or protein, is an effective way to shrink tumors and stop cancer growth. However, he believes that the healthiest, tastiest, and easiest way to restrict calories is to replace animal fats and vegetable oils with fruits, vegetables, and complex carbohydrates. It should be noted that Seyfried himself has said that this ketogenic state can also be achieved on a calorie-restricted vegan diet.

McDougall takes issue with the ketogenic diet promoters, saying that they have distorted the work of Otto Warburg to demonstrate that sugar feeds cancer. He presents research that shows that one hour after a high-fat meal, blood cells clump together and the oxygen content of the blood decreases by

20% for several hours. McDougall states: "Chronic low tissue oxygenation (hypoxia), according to Warburg, and accepted by most scientists today, causes permanent damage to cell respiration, a fundamental step for the origin of cancer cells."[13] So, according to McDougall, consuming most of your calories in the form of fats can lower your blood's oxygen levels by as much as 20% for several hours following a meal, and it's that decrease in oxygen that can stress your body's cells to where, in order to survive, they may resort to fermentation rather than respiration to create energy.

There is indeed a large body of epidemiological (population-based) studies dating from the 1970s into the present that points to the high-fat, high-meat diet of western countries as causative for many cancers and overall mortality. Often, the critics of these findings say that these studies did not control for high levels of protein, processed oils, and trans fats, all known to be harmful. But even if one is convinced by the theories of the ketogenic diet, and that sugar feeds cancer, the research about cancer cell metabolism can raise many questions.

Cancer Cell Metabolism

Cancer metabolism is a very complex subject, and researchers around the world are attempting to unravel all the complicated physiological pathways that cancer uses to sustain itself, grow, and spread. Recent research has focused on the specific metabolic pathways that cancer stem cells (CSCs) use to fuel their survival and growth. Recall that CSCs are those mother cancer cells that are the bane of conventional cancer treatment, puzzling scientists with their resistance to chemotherapy and radiation, and play a major role in metastasis.

A 2016 paper reviewed the studies that have been done on CSC metabolism in recent years.[14] The authors point to the fact that there is still no consensus on how CSCs obtain the fuel to sustain themselves, with some studies suggesting that the CSCs seem to adapt their metabolism to changes in their environment by shifting energy production from one pathway to another. They have been described as having a remarkable degree of plasticity compared to their offspring of non-stem cancer cells. Some studies have suggested that CSCs consume less glucose than ordinary cancer cells, and can even adapt to starvation, using ketones to produce energy. Researchers have also discovered that the way the CSCs obtain energy is not uniform in the different types of cancers, or even in different tumors of the same types of cancer. This paper also mentioned some of the research that looked at the changes in non-malignant cells when exposed to metabolic stresses within tumors. Some research has found that following glucose restriction, T cells, which are the body's important cancer-fighting immune cells, can develop into an immune-suppressive type of cell and actually promote tumor growth.

There is research that indicates that some types of cancer are more dependent on glucose than others. A 2017 University of Texas study identified that the two subtypes of non-small cell lung cancer— adenocarcinoma and squamous cell carcinoma—have different metabolic characteristics regarding their use of glucose. The researchers found that the squamous cell type is much more susceptible to glucose deprivation than the adenocarcinoma type. Moreover, the researchers found that squamous cell cancers of the head and neck, esophagus, and cervix also consume a lot of sugar.[15] The authors of the study did not indicate whether these findings related to CSCs as well as the cancer cells that make up the bulk of a tumor. The lead researcher of this study, Dr. Jung-whan Kim, stated that evidence is mounting that some cancers are highly dependent on sugar. His research is examining which cancers are dependent on sugar and whether cancer progression can be affected with dietary changes.

It appears that different sub-types of cancer have different susceptibilities to glucose restriction, likely making the ketogenic diet effective for some people, but not others. Until there is more science, it seems that not only is the ketogenic diet likely ineffective against the CSCs responsible for metastasis but that glucose restriction could potentially cause one's own immune cells to help fuel the cancer. Although it seems clear that this diet can shrink some tumors, it is still unknown whether it really represents a sustainable, long-term solution to cancer progression and leads to long-term remission. Certainly, eliminating refined carbohydrates and sugar is beneficial for everyone, but it is questionable if the extreme of eliminating high-carbohydrate whole foods is going to benefit every person with cancer.

In 2013, about two years before his untimely death, well-known American alternative cancer physician Nicholas Gonzalez wrote a series of eight articles concerning the ketogenic diet and those he called "ketogenic enthusiasts."[16] Gonzalez emphasized that there were no convincing human studies that suggest the diet is effective, and said, "I do have a problem when scientists go a step further, insisting in the absence of any significant human data or even impressive case histories [that] they have unraveled the mystery of cancer." Dr. Gonzalez also made the argument against the ketogenic diet for cancer based on his knowledge of the metabolic flexibility of cancer stem cells, saying that CSCs, like normal stem cells, are very flexible and able to adapt and survive in any environment.

Gerson Therapy

Likely the oldest and most well-known diet for treating cancer is the Gerson diet. There are several clinics in Tijuana that offer the Gerson Therapy, which includes an abundance of vegetable juices, supplements, and a strict dietary regimen of certain solid foods. Some of the clinics offer a more modified version of the Gerson Therapy, and many others offer elements of the therapy, such as frequent "doses" of vegetable juices and the use of coffee enemas for detoxification.

As a young medical student in the early 1900s at the University of Freiburg in Germany, the ambitious Max Gerson suffered from severe migraine headaches that sometimes left him debilitated for days. Since none of his medical school professors were able to help him with the best treatments of that era, the bright and curious young man set out to cure himself. He made dramatic changes to his diet and added supplements he thought might be helpful.

Within a few weeks the migraines disappeared. After graduation from medical school, he began prescribing the diet to his patients with migraines, with great success. One of his patients also had skin tuberculosis, and achieved a total cure on the "migraine" diet. Gerson and a renowned surgeon began a study of his diet on 460 terminal tuberculosis patients. All but four were completely cured, and Gerson became very well-known in Germany. Gerson was Jewish, and Germany was under Nazi rule at the time, so he was forced to flee. All of his siblings perished in the Holocaust, but he managed to escape to France and eventually found his way to New York, where he passed the medical boards and set up a practice in Manhattan.

Although it was not Gerson's intention to treat cancer, cancer patients came to him, desperate for a cure. He began quietly treating them, despite the risks of deviating from the standard of cancer treatment of the 1940s. And he did suffer the consequences, despite presenting evidence of his cancer cures. The idea that diet could affect health was considered completely radical, but Gerson continued to publish articles in the few journals that were receptive to his work. Eventually Gerson lost his membership in the New York Medical Society and was prohibited from publishing his work in peer-reviewed medical journals. Gerson died in 1959, in New York, and there are many who believe he was poisoned by an enemy within the medical establishment. Gerson had been a long-time friend of Albert Schweitzer, the great humanitarian, physician, and 1952 Nobel Peace Prize winner, whose eulogy of Gerson read: "I see in him one of the most eminent geniuses in the history of medicine. Many of his basic ideas have been adopted without having his name connected with them. Yet, he has achieved more than seemed possible under adverse conditions. He leaves a legacy which commands attention and which will assure him his due place. Those whom he has cured will now attest to the truth of his ideas."[17]

The Gerson treatment for cancer and other chronic diseases was eventually brought to Mexico by Gerson's daughter Charlotte. Although not a doctor herself, she was very involved with her father's practice of medicine and the Gerson Therapy. The Gerson Institute, established by Charlotte Gerson, has a clinic in Playas de Tijuana, as well as in Hungary, that offers the classic Gerson treatment. Other clinics in the Tijuana area offer the Gerson treatment, and some of their medical directors worked with Charlotte Gerson in the past. These clinics have added other therapies to the Gerson approach, convinced that this was Dr. Gerson's intention. (I visited these clinics in

Playas de Tijuana and Rosarito, and they will be described further on in this chapter.)

The Gerson treatment involves flooding the body daily with nutrients from fifteen to twenty pounds of organically grown fruits and vegetables. Fresh raw juices are consumed up to thirteen times per day. Raw and cooked solid foods are a part of the treatment, with the diet being very low fat, low protein, and low sodium. The diet includes cooked vegetables, oatmeal, potatoes, modest amounts of fruits, and a small amount of flax oil in addition to all the raw vegetable juices. Multiple coffee enemas each day are an integral part of the Gerson Therapy, considered essential for detoxification.

Gerson wrote prolifically about the physiological rationale for his treatment, and like physician and researcher Otto Warburg, he zeroed in on the function of the mitochondria within the cells. Unlike Warburg, he focused on the balance of sodium and potassium within cells and its influence on the production of energy by the mitochondria. Gar Hildenbrand, a long-term advocate for the Gerson Therapy and current president of the Gerson Research Organization, wrote a paper based on his lectures about the physiological mechanisms that are responsible for the therapeutic value of this dietary approach for cancer.[18]

Hildenbrand compares the mitochondria to the industrial city of a cell, responsible for producing the energy that the cell needs to function correctly. He states that when a cell has lost potassium and gained sodium and has swollen with water, the mitochondria's function is shut down, and energy in the form of ATP (adenosine triphosphate) cannot be made to correct the imbalance. One of the ways the Gerson Therapy aims to correct this basic dysfunction and increase energy production is by restricting sodium and protein and supplementing with potassium. Gerson eliminated protein from the diet for a limited period of time as he found that doing so enhanced the desired effect of reducing the amount of sodium within the cells. According to Hildenbrand, there is also evidence that short-term protein restriction enhances immunity, and he points to the research of Dr. Robert Good, former director of the Sloan-Kettering Institute for Cancer Research.

Calorie restriction is another feature of the Gerson Therapy, but is entirely different from the calorie restriction of the ketogenic diet. In the Gerson Therapy, calories from proteins and fats are restricted, with only about 90 calories a day from fats, and the diet provides most of its calories in the form of carbohydrates. After about six to eight weeks on the diet, supplemental protein is provided. Another focus of the classic Gerson Therapy is the supplementation with iodine and thyroid hormone, which according to Hildenbrand, signals the mitochondria to multiply and increase the production of energy in the form of ATP.

In a nutshell, the Gerson Therapy involves sodium, protein, and calorie restriction, along with potassium and thyroid supplementation. The very high degree of natural enzymes, antioxidants, and phytochemicals from vegetable juice also contributes to the diet's anti-cancer effects. (This will be explored further on, when looking at why all diets that target cancer include large amounts of vegetables.) There are numerous reports of the Gerson Therapy being successful at inducing cancer remission in people, even in those with advanced cancers. Several books have been written by people who have been cured of cancer using the Gerson approach. Others have reported feeling very weak after being on the Gerson Therapy for a length of time. Some have felt that adhering to the diet is so labor- and time-intensive that it consumed their entire life.

It is difficult to implement the Gerson Therapy without help and qualified guidance. It is very laborious and expensive to make the volume of juices required for the diet. The Gerson Institute states that six hundred pounds of organic produce is needed for the full protocol for one month, which costs well over a thousand dollars a month at today's prices. The cost of the necessary supplements and organic coffee for the enemas is estimated to cost another few hundred dollars per month. Treatment at one of the Gerson clinics is typically three weeks, and it is usually required to bring a companion to learn the therapeutic program, as the Gerson doctors recognize that it is too much work for the patient to do without assistance at home.

Enzyme Therapy

Although enzyme therapy is not a diet per se, it is often considered a part of nutritional protocols as well as a metabolic approach to cancer. Many of the A/I doctors in Tijuana, as well as in the United States and Germany, use large doses of enzymes, taken orally, for the treatment of cancer. Enzymes are biological proteins that are abundant in plants and also produced by the body during digestion. Enzymes act as catalysts, accelerating chemical reactions, and are essential to digesting proteins, fats, and carbohydrates. Cancer cells are believed to have a fibrin/protein coating that renders them invisible to the natural killer cells of the immune system, with the result that natural killer cells view the cancer as normal, rather than mutated cells that should be eliminated. Enzymes, especially pancreatic enzymes, are capable of dissolving this fibrin coating so that cancer cells can be recognized as mutated and harmful by the immune cells and destroyed.[19] It has been theorized that the high level of animal protein contained in the diets of industrialized societies creates a deficit in the supply of enzymes in the body, with less available to dissolve the fibrin coating of cancer cells.

It has been reported that when tumors are exposed to various drugs in the lab to determine their effectiveness, the tumor is first treated with enzymes to dissolve the protein coating.[20] This could explain why some drugs may be effective at killing cancer in a petri dish, but are not as effective within the human body. It would seem safe and reasonable for enzymes to be advised prior to treatment with chemotherapy and other drugs, but that is not a typical practice in conventional cancer treatment. This ability of enzymes to make cancer cells more vulnerable could also partly explain why a diet that is abundant in fruits and vegetables is often protective against cancer, although it is the pancreatic enzymes that are believed to be the most powerful for cancer prevention and treatment.

The late New York physician Nicholas Gonzalez relied on pancreatic enzymes as a component of his cancer treatment protocols, and he was known for helping even Stage IV pancreatic cancer patients achieve remission using individually prescribed nutritional protocols, high doses of enzymes, supplements, and detoxification. In Gonzalez's presentations,[21] articles,[22] and posthumously published book *Nutrition and the Autonomic Nervous System*,[23] Gonzalez refers to the work of Scottish biologist John Beard, a researcher at the University of Edinburgh who wrote *The Enzyme Treatment of Cancer*, published in 1911.

The research of Beard that informs the Gonzalez protocol, as well as the protocols of other physicians, is intriguing. The primary theory concerns the existence and function of cells called trophoblasts. Trophoblasts are cells that provide nutrients to an embryo and develop into the placenta. They are formed during the initial stage of pregnancy and are the first cells to differentiate from the fertilized egg. Trophoblasts share three important characteristics with cancer cells: 1) they can divide very quickly; 2) they invade maternal tissue; and 3) they generate their own blood supply.

Beard reasoned that the trophoblast initially behaves as any growing tumor would, but at some predetermined point, the placenta transforms from a highly invasive, rapidly growing, blood vessel-producing, tumor-like tissue to the non-invasive, non-proliferating mature organ. Beard claimed that the only difference between the placenta and a malignant growth is that the placenta knows when to stop growing while tumors do not. Beard spent years studying this transformation from an invasive aggressive tissue to the stable and nurturing tissues of the placenta. What Beard eventually discovered is that at the precise time the trophoblasts cease to be aggressive is the very time when the fetus begins to secrete its own pancreatic enzymes. In animal studies and in clinical work with cancer patients, Beard proved that pancreatic enzymes could attack and destroy cancerous tumors.

Like that of many scientists who were before their time and thought "outside the box," Beard's work was mocked and belittled by the media and scientific community. Although there were physicians and scientists who were supportive of Beard and his theories, according to Gonzalez, "Interest in Beard's thesis gradually petered out, largely due to the excitement over the potential of radiation treatment for cancer, and when he passed away in 1924, he died frustrated, angry, and ignored, his therapy already considered no more than a historical oddity."[24]

The Raw Vegan, Plant-Based, and Mediterranean Diets

There are many, many people with cancer who attribute their cure or remission to following an initially raw, strictly plant-based diet, consuming liberal quantities of vegetable juice and eliminating refined sugar and processed foods, a diet similar to what my mother adopted. Chris Wark, a popular blogger and cancer coach, was diagnosed with Stage IIIC colon cancer in 2003. He refused chemotherapy after surgery and used natural therapies and a vegan diet, including sixty-four ounces of vegetable juice daily, to recover from cancer. His website (chrisbeatcancer.com) features many video interviews of people like him who radically changed their diets and defied the odds, thriving after even advanced cancer diagnoses. There are many other longtime survivors of cancer who followed and recommend a similar diet, including physician Lorraine Day, who healed her own breast cancer without conventional treatment and developed an in-depth protocol. To my knowledge, there is no evidence-based proof of this approach, no clinical trials or formal studies, no academic articles that I can present that show the effectiveness of this approach. As with the various alternative therapies, it would not be considered ethical to withhold the standard of care from patients in order to evaluate the efficacy of nutritional approaches to cancer.

Although there may not be academic literature that supports the effectiveness of a mostly raw plant-based diet for treating cancer, there is no lack of scientific research regarding the benefits of fruits, vegetables, and herbs against cancer. There are also several studies showing a decrease in recurrence and mortality for some cancers by following a whole-foods plant-based diet.[25] There is an abundance of academic literature that suggests the Mediterranean diet is associated with a reduced risk of overall cancer incidence and mortality.[26] The Mediterranean diet consists of the high consumption of vegetables, fruits, nuts, legumes, unprocessed cereals, fish, and a high ratio of unsaturated fats (mostly olive oil) to saturated fats. Meats and dairy are considered detrimental and are very limited in a classic Mediterranean diet.

What's the Problem with Animal Protein?

There is an abundance of research that supports the idea that minimizing or eliminating animal protein is beneficial for cancer and other chronic, degenerative diseases. The cancer-promoting qualities of meat are attributed to high amounts of heme iron (specifically red meats), methionine, and insulin-like growth factor (IGF-1). These three substances are present in meat, even when the animals are grass fed/free range or organically raised.

Heme iron is iron that is obtained from animal sources, whereas non-heme iron derives from plant sources. Although heme iron is better absorbed than non-heme iron, many studies suggest that high levels of heme iron contribute not only to cancer but stroke, metabolic syndrome, and cardiac events. Several studies have suggested that the heme iron in red meat contributes to cancers of the breast,[27] pancreas,[28] colon,[29] and lung,[30] as well as overall cancer risk and progression.[31]

Methionine is an amino acid that is a building block for proteins, essential for cell development and growth. The foods highest in methionine are animal products, with a vegan diet representing the most methionine-restricted diet. Rapidly dividing cancer cells require more methionine than normal cells, and several studies[32] have shown the effect of methionine restriction on cancer cells. Methionine restriction causes cancer cells to stop growing and dividing, and increases the rate of cancer cell death, decreasing or stopping metastasis. These studies discovered that many types of cancer require methionine to grow and divide, including the most common solid and blood cancers.

One of the more controversial arguments for decreasing animal protein is found in the studies regarding a hormone called insulin-like growth factor, or IGF-1. IGF-1 is instrumental in normal growth during childhood and puberty, but in adulthood can promote abnormal growth in the form of proliferation, metastasis, and invasion of cancer. Research has suggested that high animal protein intake raises IGF-1 levels[33] and those with certain cancers have been found to have higher than average levels of IGF-1. Low protein intake in those under age sixty-five has been suggested to be responsible for a major reduction in IGF-1, cancer, and overall mortality. In older adults, however, higher protein intake may be protective.

Although there are many studies that examine the role of IGF-1 and cancer risk and progression,[34] the strongest association appears to be in prostate and breast cancer, although it has been implicated in other cancers. The association seems to be the strongest when high intake of dairy products and/or obesity is also a factor. It continues to be an area of active research interest, with some clinicians feeling strongly that the higher IGF-1 levels found in those with cancer are causative and a result of a high animal protein diet. There are others who are more cautious, pointing out that low IGF-1 levels are associated with risks of cardiovascular disease and dementia.

Since there are many other reasons to decrease animal protein and adopt a largely plant-based diet, I don't believe that the mixed opinions about IGF-1 and cancer risk and progression are particularly relevant. It is well known that conventionally produced meat and dairy foods in the U.S. generally contain high levels of antibiotics and growth hormones, so unless one can obtain free-range or organically raised animal products, these substances also contribute to the detrimental health effects of animal protein. In the case of dairy, even the milk from organically fed, free-range dairy cows is likely to contain excessive amounts of estrogen and other hormones. The dairy cows of commercial milk production, whether organic or not, produce milk throughout their numerous pregnancies.

Processed and red meats are believed to be the most detrimental to health. A study of over half a million people, which looked at all meat consumption, concluded that red and processed meat intake is associated with increases in total mortality, cancer mortality, and cardiovascular disease mortality.[35] The evidence that red and processed meat contributes to cancer incidence is so strong that WHO, the World Health Organization, has issued an official statement cautioning about their consumption.[36] Processed meat is classified as carcinogenic to humans, based on sufficient evidence that its consumption causes colorectal cancer. Red meat is classified as probably carcinogenic to humans based on limited evidence that the consumption of red meat causes cancer in humans and strong evidence supporting a carcinogenic effect.

The Anti-Cancer Benefits of Plants

So what is so great about consuming mostly plants? What do fruits and vegetables possess that have an anti-cancer effect? In addition to being rich in a variety of enzymes and antioxidants, substances that neutralize free-radical damage and protect cells, plant foods contain numerous phytonutrients. Phytonutrients, sometimes referred to as phytochemicals, are known to have specific actions that contribute to preventing and healing cancer. Many of these have familiar names, such as beta carotene, resveratrol, and lycopene, but there are many others that are not as widely known. Many phytonutrients have antioxidant properties but also have a variety of anti-carcinogenic properties. For example, blueberry extract has been shown to decrease the growth and metastatic potential of cells associated with breast cancer in mice, and in laboratory cell cultures.[37]

Numerous studies over the past twenty years have found that the various antioxidants and phytonutrients in fruits and vegetables are protective against cancer and other diseases. There is also research that suggests that a combination of fruits and vegetables have a synergistic effect, and are far more powerful than a single phytonutrient alone. One study treated two different types of breast cancer cells with a six-phytonutrient extract cocktail, and also using individual extracts, to determine how powerful a combination might be.[38] The phytonutrients were supplied to the cancer cells at concentrations similar to the levels found when humans consumed these compounds from food. The study found that when tested individually, the phytonutrient compounds demonstrated minimal anticancer effect, but when all six compounds were given together, they slowed cancer cell growth by more than 80% and triggered apoptosis—programmed cell death.

Many of the studies showing the benefit of consuming phytonutrients have been done in the lab, and occasionally with mice. An exception was a recent study done with men who had localized prostate cancer. A group of men took a supplement called POMI-T, which contains broccoli, turmeric, pomegranate, and green tea, while a similar group of men took a placebo. After the six-month trial, 46% of the men in the supplement group had PSA (prostate specific antigen) levels that were lower or stable, while only 14% of the men who took the placebo had lower or stable levels. In addition, the men who took the supplement had a median rise in PSA levels of 14.7%, while those who took the placebo had a rise of 78.5%.[39]

One beneficial feature of many phytonutrients is their ability to inhibit angiogenesis. Angiogenesis is the process by which new blood vessels are formed, which are essential to the growth and spread of cancer. A cancerous growth cannot grow more than about two millimeters (less than 0.08 inches) without a blood supply. Many of the newer cancer drugs impede angiogenesis, with Avastin being one of the more frequently used anti-angiogenesis drugs.

Physician and researcher William Li is the president and medical director of the Angiogenesis Foundation, whose stated mission is to improve global health by advancing angiogenesis-based medicine, diet, and lifestyle. Li has done research on the ability of certain foods to inhibit angiogenesis, studying the anti-angiogenesis properties of common foods and comparing them with the actions of anti-angiogenic drugs. In his research, some phytonutrients outperformed some of the drugs, and many phytonutrients generated strong anti-angiogenesis activity that approached the degree found in the drugs.[40]

Common foods that have been found to inhibit angiogenesis include a long list of fruits like grapes, berries, pineapple, apple, citrus, and tomatoes, among many other foods, including garlic, parsley, and broccoli. Black teas, green teas, and turmeric were the phytonutrient-containing substances found to possess the highest anti-angiogenesis properties in his research. In addition, Li found that combining varieties of black and green tea had a synergistic effect, becoming more potent against angiogenesis than one variety of tea alone. Again, this points to the value of combining plant foods in an anti-cancer diet.

Li mentions a Harvard study of 79,000 men that looked at dietary habits and prostate cancer. Men who consumed two to three servings of cooked tomatoes per week had a 40–50% reduced risk of developing prostate cancer. Furthermore, in those who did develop prostate cancer, those who ate the most tomato products had fewer blood vessels feeding their cancer. The research of Li and his colleagues suggests that an anti-angiogenic diet could provide a safe, widely available, and novel strategy for preventing cancer.[41]

Another process by which the various phytonutrients can inhibit cancer progression is a form of apoptosis, often called "cell suicide." Apoptosis is how the body eliminates damaged cells, yet in cancer this process is inhibited, allowing mutated cells to survive. Numerous phytonutrients have demonstrated an ability to induce apoptosis of cancer cells.[42] These include green tea, turmeric, numerous fruits, capsaicin (hot pepper), ginger, garlic, and onion, to name but a few. Cruciferous vegetables (those in the broccoli family) contain not one but two phytonutrients known to encourage apoptosis of cancer cells.

There are few drugs that effectively target and kill cancer stem cells (CSCs), yet numerous substances in plants have been identified to have such power. A 2015 study reviewed the literature regarding the properties of various phytonutrients against cancer stem cells, stating: "Recent studies evaluating natural products against CSC support the epidemiological evidence linking plant-based diets with reduced malignancy rates."[43] The authors stated that many natural products tested have demonstrated the ability to modulate the pathways responsible for CSC function as well as inhibition. The review listed the top twenty-five substances active against CSCs, including compounds found in green tea, ginger, turmeric, berries, grapes, carrots, tomatoes, leafy greens, cruciferous vegetables, onions, and black pepper, as well as other less commonly used substances like guggul, feverfew, corn lily, and Chinese skullcap.[44]

Although many of the studies demonstrating the anticancer effects of various plant foods involve using plant extracts in the laboratory rather than whole foods, the whole plant has benefits far beyond its chemical composition, and the consumption of whole foods is far superior to taking handfuls of supplements. Plant foods have a vast array of vitamins, minerals, and fiber, all contributing to a decrease in the inflammation that is often a precursor to cancer initiation and recurrence. Recall that a healthy gut microbiome is essential to a highly functioning immune system, and is reliant on the fiber from plant foods. Supplements may have a role, but do not replace the powerful nutritional medicine of a plant-based diet.

It is estimated that only 5–10% of cancer is genetic, while the remaining

90–95% is the result of environmental factors. Environmental factors include alcohol, obesity, tobacco, and infections, but none of these categories top the estimated 35% of environmental causation by diet.[45] For those who have been consuming a standard American diet for some time, a radical change to a whole-foods plant-based diet can be an extremely powerful therapy, regardless of whether one chooses A/I (alternative/integrative) or conventional cancer treatment. Even the American Cancer Society has spoken out about the influence of diet on cancer incidence and cites studies that show improved cancer survival by adopting a plant-based diet. It calls for oncologists to integrate this nutritional information into their patient care. "The oncologist and the oncology care team now stand at a unique interface—delivering acute care aimed at a life-threatening disease while at the same time readying the patient for a long and healthy life free of comorbidity. Good nutrition and a physically active lifestyle are central to both pursuits, and it is becoming increasingly apparent that these factors need to be routinely integrated into the delivery of optimal cancer care."[46]

Arguably, the biggest decision for those with cancer who are prepared to make a radical dietary change is whether to adopt the ketogenic diet or a mostly vegan version of a plant-based diet supplemented with vegetable juices. The information available is abundant and convincing for both strategies, with equally qualified and respected doctors and scientists promoting one over the other. In one camp, carbs are "bad" and fat is "good." The other camp makes a convincing argument for just the opposite.

Another debate concerns the effect of the different diets on the microbiome, and conflicting opinions abound. The two sides agree only that protein should be limited, processed foods and refined sugar should be eliminated, and many vegetables should be consumed. The varying arguments about which diet is best for people with cancer are quite scientific and convincing, bringing it right down to the tiny mitochondria and how they function on a low-fat or a low-carb diet. The obvious place to start is to make those changes on which both camps agree, while doing one's own research and ultimately making the choice that feels right for the individual. In the beginning, choosing the nutrition plan that feels the most doable, and creates the least amount of stress, may be the more beneficial choice in the big picture of cancer recovery.

There are many food-based supplements and herbs known to be extremely valuable for those with cancer, regardless of what type of treatment is chosen. Although a discussion of these is beyond the scope of this book, there is one supplement that is relevant in the context of deciding between a ketogenic diet or a whole-foods plant-based diet. Avemar, a fermented wheat germ extract, is a very well-studied supplement that is known to significantly interfere with the glucose metabolism of cancer cells, in addition to its other anti-cancer actions.[47] Avemar is likely a good choice for all cancer patients, but may provide particular reassurance to those who need more calories than a ketogenic or raw vegan diet, but are concerned or convinced that the glucose in unrefined carbohydrates may fuel their cancer.

Between the extremes of the raw vegan diet, the ketogenic diet, and the Gerson Therapy, most of the physicians of the A/I clinics that I visited in Mexico recommend a more moderate approach to the diet for their patients. Although all offer and encourage fresh vegetable juices, the diets more closely resemble a moderate plant-based diet with an abundance of vegetables, small amounts of animal protein, unprocessed whole grains, and small quantities of fruit and healthy fats. With the exception of the doctors of the Gerson Therapy clinics, the doctors that I spoke to about their recommended diets unanimously view a patient's diet as an integral component of a new lifestyle that contributes to health and supports the medical treatments. Most of the clinics also include enzyme therapy in their prescribed treatments. Other than the Gerson-therapy-based clinics, all of the individual clinics have their own particular nutritional philosophies and degrees of stringency toward the diets provided or recommended. (These will be described in clinic descriptions in subsequent chapters.)

Part 2

This next part of the book changes gears and takes the reader along on my travels in Tijuana. In addition to a description of the clinics I visited, the stories of some of the patients I met, and a bit of history about the Tijuana alternative cancer clinic phenomenon, these chapters also address the questions that a potential patient frequently has:

Is Tijuana a safe place to go?
Will these clinics/doctors really help me?
What is the cost?
Does health insurance cover any of the cost?
Are the doctors qualified?
How do I choose the best clinic for me?

CHAPTER 7

Arriving in Tijuana
International Bio-Care and the Bio-Medical Center

For my first visit to Tijuana, I had planned on a guided tour of five of the clinics through the Cancer Control Society, but the bus tour that was to commence in Los Angeles and San Diego was canceled due to a lack of participants. I decided to organize my own tour, traveling alone, with my rusty college Spanish and a thirst to satisfy my curiosity about these clinics, doctors, and the patients who go to them. I contacted some of the clinics prior to my trip and scheduled appointments with those who were willing to have me visit.

Although many patients take a private van from the San Diego airport to Tijuana, I took the hour-long trip on the San Diego trolley to its last stop, right at the border crossing in San Ysidro, California. I admit I felt a little bit intimidated as I prepared to leave the United States and enter Mexico. The area looked a bit seamy, but I felt only mildly uncomfortable and confidently walked to the immigration entrance without incident. Even on a Sunday morning, it was a busy and frenetic place, with the neon signs of money changers and fast-food places, buses, trolleys, and taxis coming and going, and so many people arriving from Mexico. A long uphill walk along a fenced concrete path brought me to the Mexican customs building, where I presented my passport and sailed through the quick and cursory paperwork and security screening. Another lengthy walk, this time downhill along a narrow concrete ramp, took me to the taxi area, past young men tending old wooden carts and offering to assist me with my luggage, and women sitting on the ground with babies, asking for money. This would be the only time I encountered anyone asking for a handout in my travels in the Tijuana area. A multitude of bright yellow taxicabs waited at the end of the ramp, and although the first, rather irritable driver refused my offer of twelve dollars to take me to the beach suburb of Playas de Tijuana, another friendly and engaging young man was happy to take me. Although I spoke with them in Spanish, the taxi drivers seem to know enough English to serve the many *gringos* who crossed daily.

The land border arrival area in Tijuana is in a very busy commercial district, and it looked much like other cities, if a bit ragged and run down. The fifteen-minute drive to Playas, as the beach suburb of Playas de Tijuana is called, took me along the main highway past some neighborhoods that were shockingly poor and derelict, with a variety of shack-like dwellings flowing down hillsides that boasted panoramic views of the border area and prosperous San Diego beyond. Arriving in Playas, I found a busy, thriving area with some beautiful homes and modern shopping centers, although the roads were cracked and potholed, like many in Tijuana. Settling into the comfortable and peaceful Dali Suites hotel, built around gardens and secured by a tall wall and locked gate, I prepared for my first week of exploring Tijuana and visiting clinics.

Later that day, I walked all around Playas, through commercial and residential areas and along the lively ocean boardwalk lined with cafés and restaurants, where families gathered in the evenings and on weekends. I was politely ignored by the locals, which was my experience during all of my travels in Tijuana and Playas, unless I asked for help finding my way. I went grocery shopping at a large modern supermarket and was surprised at how similar it was to those in the United States. I discovered that businesses accepted U.S. dollars as well as Mexican pesos, and I noticed that Mexican customers carried both currencies in their wallets. I used a credit card at the supermarket and never did get around to changing dollars into pesos during my first stay in Tijuana.

The next morning, the hotel management called a favored taxi driver to take me to my first appointment. Felipe picked me up right on time, and in addition to being a very pleasant and jovial older man, he spoke decent

English. As we chatted in a mix of English and Spanish, Felipe wound his way through the frenetic traffic of Tijuana, arriving at the **International Bio-Care Hospital** on time for the appointment I had scheduled a week or two prior. IBC, as the International Bio-Care Health and Wellness Center is called, was established in 1996 by Dr. Rodrigo Rodriguez, and is a well-known and respected integrative cancer treatment hospital.

I had heard positive feedback about IBC from a few former patients or family members of patients. One of the most interesting stories was told to me by Maebell Beard, the wife of a patient who had been treated at IBC many years earlier.

Maebell's husband Edwin was an engineer, a very logical, intelligent, left-brain sort of man who was enjoying his mid-life years in Phoenix with Maebell when he was diagnosed with prostate cancer. A man of science, he sought out the best oncologist and cancer center in the area that his research could uncover. He underwent surgery to remove his prostate, and, later, his testicles, had radiation treatment, and was glad that chemotherapy was not advised. Despite undergoing what he considered to be the most up-to-date, evidence-based treatments available, the cancer eventually spread to his bones and his prognosis became very poor. Ed and Maebell were told there was nothing more that could be done for Ed, that he was now considered "terminal," and that he should get his affairs in order and enjoy his remaining days.

Although Maebell has always been a strong and optimistic woman, she was devastated, and dreaded the thought of watching her life partner and best friend suffer and wither away like Barbara, an acquaintance of Maebell's who had been treated for lymphoma. Each time Maebell saw her, Barbara was thinner, weaker, and sicklier looking. In fact, because she hadn't seen or heard from Barbara in several years, Maebell had presumed she'd passed away.

Barbara, however, had not passed away. One day when Maebell was out doing errands, a woman stopped to say hello to her, and it took Maebell a moment to recognize her. Maebell was shocked. Barbara appeared strong and vibrant as she greeted Maebell and inquired after Maebell and her family. When Maebell told Barbara about Ed's terminal diagnosis, Barbara shared her story of recovery from lymphoma, receiving treatment, she said, at a clinic in Tijuana that provided several therapies that were not part of the treatment recommended in Phoenix. Barbara offered to meet with Ed to share her experiences and what she had learned at the International Bio-Care Hospital in Tijuana.

Although Ed was as surprised as Maebell to discover that Barbara was alive, and he agreed to speak with her, he was very skeptical that any doctor in Tijuana could offer anything more effective than what the top oncologist at an esteemed cancer center could offer. He believed that if there were indeed better treatments, his doctor would surely know about them. Maebell disagreed and encouraged Ed to go to Tijuana for treatment, but his resistance was reinforced by relatives who argued that he would be totally crazy to go to Mexico.

Still highly skeptical, but wanting to placate his wife, he agreed to travel to Tijuana and consult the doctors at International Bio-Care. Ed met with Dr. Romero to discuss his case and learn about the recommended treatment options. Ed was impressed with what he saw and heard, and decided to try the unconventional treatment despite the continuing negative pressure from other members of his family.

Ed went for three weeks of treatments and followed his after-care plan at home, which involved a radical change in his usual diet. He returned to the clinic six months later for a re-evaluation and more treatments, and just like after the first three weeks of treatments, he found himself feeling better than he had in years. Curiously, Maebell noticed that Ed always returned from Mexico with an unusual odor, and Maebell thought it was likely the result of the detoxification treatments clearing out the ill effects of years of a standard American processed-food diet.

Three months after his second round of treatment in Tijuana, Ed returned to his Phoenix oncologist for a bone scan. His oncologist expressed astonishment that there were no new areas of cancer. Moreover, the previously identified bone lesions were barely visible on the scan.

Maebell admitted to feeling disappointed, as she had anticipated the scan showing that all of the cancer would now be gone. According to Maebell, the oncologist said, "The tumor is dying." He added, "I can't condone what you are doing or I will lose my job," but he did not advise Ed to stop doing what he was doing.

Feeling quite optimistic, Ed stuck with his treatment program religiously, following the diet and taking the prescribed supplements. Another three months later, Ed returned to his oncologist for another bone scan. This time, the oncologist was very happy and only a bit less astonished to report that no evidence of cancer was found. Maebell and Ed were elated and very grateful.

Maebell and Ed became active advocates of alternative and integrative cancer treatment, hosting informational support groups for people with cancer in their community. It was not until twenty-three cancer-free years later that Maebell finally said goodbye to her husband when Ed passed away from complications of Alzheimer's disease, in 2014.

The International Bio-Care Hospital where Ed had received treatment would be the first clinic I visited during my initial trip to Tijuana, and I met with Dr. Romero, who had been Ed's doctor all those years ago.

IBC was located on a narrow street on the outer edge of the Zona Rio district of Tijuana, the area where many of the clinics are located, and Felipe and I found the well-kept and clearly marked building easily. A short walk across a pretty tiled garden patio led to a reception area with modern and professional furnishings, just like many health facilities in the United States. I was escorted to the office of Dr. Romero, a physician who had worked at IBC for many years. Although I had stated my intention for the visit when I had scheduled the appointment, Dr. Romero thought I was a potential patient. Nevertheless, after some inquiry into the purpose of my visit, she was quite willing to speak with me and explain the therapies offered and the treatment philosophy.

Dr. Romero said that most of the patients who come to IBC are in the later stages of the disease and have already undergone conventional cancer treatment that failed. Dr. Romero endorsed the need for some conventional treatments and described IBC as a very integrative cancer hospital, applying the best approaches from both worlds. Dr. Romero stressed that it is not one specific treatment that produces successful results; rather, it is the totality of the whole program that restores health, detoxifies the body, and targets the cancer.

After meeting with Dr. Romero, I was given a lengthy tour of the facility by one of the hospital's employees, who was very welcoming, professional, informative, and spoke perfect English. A large dining room was located next to the reception area and business office, and I was offered a glass of green juice from a pitcher that had been prepared for the patients' breakfast.

As I sipped my juice, I was shown the various treatment areas along a hallway that included the office of an acupuncturist who was described as an excellent healer. I was told that acupuncture is not included in the basic cancer program, but is available and encouraged, as are the services of a chiropractor who also has an office in the building. At the end of the hallway was a large intravenous therapy treatment area, where a few people were receiving therapies. This bright and spacious room opened onto a large outdoor terrace with seating areas and exercise equipment.

We walked down to the lower level, where the patient rooms are located. This area looked like a standard hospital floor, plain but clean, with a central nursing station and standard hospital beds. My guide told me that IBC is able to care for patients who are not capable of self-care or medically stable, and that in addition to 24-hour nursing care, an on-call physician is in the building at all times.

I was taken to see several cottage-style apartments located next to the hospital building where outpatients or families of inpatients stay. This area felt like a little village of adjacent attractive and clean apartments, ranging from one to three bedrooms. I was told that IBC serves many Amish patients, who tend to travel with a large family group, making the apartments ideal for them. The largest, a spacious three-bedroom dwelling, cost $110 per night.

My guide said that IBC has treated patients from all over the United States, Canada, and other countries, and I was surprised to learn that IBC has had many patients who are licensed American physicians. I was told that most patients are referred by word of mouth, but there are some doctors in the United States who quietly refer cancer patients to IBC.

The last stop on my tour was the clinic's business office, where I met with

Socorra, a woman who has been the financial coordinator of the hospital since its inception. She was very upfront and informative about the costs of treatment at IBC, and she told me that many patients get some of their costs reimbursed by their health insurance companies. She mentioned that Blue Cross Blue Shield seemed to be the association that patients had the most success with. My meeting with Socorra concluded my visit, and confirmed my perception that IBC is a very organized, efficient, and professional facility.

(I visited IBC for a second time on the Cancer Control Society bus tour of clinics during a later trip to Tijuana. During that visit, the founder and medical director, Dr. Rodriguez, gave a presentation that included his views about the growing problem of cancer in the United States, and the importance of nutrition as a cancer prevention strategy. He also spoke to us about the emotional and spiritual aspects of recovering from cancer, and expressed his views about stress as a major contributor to illness. Although I enjoyed meeting Dr. Rodriguez and hearing his presentation, I found that my earlier private visit offered a more satisfying and detailed glimpse into the workings of the hospital.)

IBC offers a variety of cancer therapies based on an assessment of each person's needs. IBC's treatment philosophy is to restore the best possible health through nutrition, rest, and exercise, while detoxifying the body, regulating the immune system, and targeting cancer. Both alternative and conventional modalities are used against the cancer, including hyperthermia, dendritic cell vaccines, oxygen therapies, ultraviolet blood irradiation, and a variety of intravenous therapies that include laetrile, vitamin C, and various supplements. Low-dose chemotherapy is done in combination with hyperthermia when indicated. Nutrition is a major focus, and the dietary department serves a mostly organic, plant-based diet with only small amounts of chicken and fish. Vegetable juices are encouraged and available throughout the day. Nutrition and supplements, coffee enemas, and chelation are prescribed to address detoxification needs.

IBC serves inpatients in the hospital that provides twenty-four-hour nursing care and physician availability. Companions are welcome to stay in the patient's room. For those returning for follow-up visits, accommodations are available adjacent to *the hospital. In 2016 the cost of a three-week inpatient treatment program was $27,000, which included two hyperthermia treatments, various intravenous therapies, and dendritic cell vaccines to take home for self-administration. Room and board for a companion, and transportation from the San Diego airport, is also included in this price. Other, more specialized therapies, such as autologous stem cells or live cell therapy, are not included in the base price. Credit cards are accepted. For more information, visit http://www.biocarehospital.com.*

✲

On the second day of this trip, I visited the American-owned-and-operated **Bio-Medical Center**, also known as the **Hoxsey Clinic**, where Marie Carlson had received treatment for breast cancer. Felipe didn't require any directions as it was well known to him, and he has taken many people to the clinic over the years. I was invited, as are other interested American doctors and nurses, to spend up to a week at the clinic. They required that I send my résumé and R.N. license number, and that I schedule the visit in advance. Before going, I knew that the Bio-Medical Center was a very special place, with a long and colorful history, and I was looking forward to my visit.

The Bio-Medical Center has the distinction of being the first, and likely the most visited, alternative cancer clinic in Tijuana, thanks to Harry Hoxsey and Mildred Nelson. In 1946, Mildred Nelson, a feisty, straight-talking Texan and registered nurse, was horrified that her parents were going to the controversial Hoxsey Clinic in Dallas for treatment of her mother's Stage IV cancer. At the time, the Hoxsey Clinic was quite famous for curing cancer, using the herbal formula that was passed down to the self-educated layman Harry Hoxsey by his veterinarian grandfather. When Mildred's father asked her to come with them, Mildred flatly refused. "We are going to see the best there is," she stated. "Just forget that. You are not going to see a damn quack!"

Mildred's parents insisted that they were going, with or without Mildred, so Mildred decided to accompany them to investigate the "quackery" herself. Despite her skepticism, Harry Hoxsey offered Mildred a job, and Mildred accepted for the sole purpose of disproving the therapy and revealing Harry Hoxsey as the fraud and quack she believed him to be. However, rather than disproving the therapy, Mildred became convinced that the herbal formulas were saving lives and sparing people the suffering of the very toxic and aggressive therapies of conventional medicine at that time. Mildred eventually became Hoxsey's chief nurse. Among the many cures she witnessed was that of her mother, who lived to a ripe old age and outlived many of her doctors in their hometown.

The various medical authorities were constantly harassing Harry Hoxsey, often putting him in jail for practicing medicine without a license, despite the numerous positive testimonials from his patients. The dramatic legal battles that Hoxsey fought are chronicled in his book *You Don't Have to Die*, including stories about how his patients would surround the jail, demanding his release. The Texas Medical Board, as well as the president of the newly formed American Medical Association, applied tremendous pressure to have the clinic closed, and in 1960, they finally succeeded.

After the FDA closed down the Hoxsey Clinic, Harry Hoxsey remained in Texas and asked Mildred to reopen the center in Tijuana, giving it a different name to avoid attention from the government. The Bio-Medical Center, the oldest alternative cancer treatment clinic in Tijuana, was established by Mildred in 1963 in a hilltop villa, overlooking the city of Tijuana. For over fifty years, the Bio-Medical Center has thrived, serving people with cancer from all over the globe. Mildred passed away in 2014, leaving her sister, Liz Jonas, to carry on the legacy of Harry Hoxsey and the Hoxsey herbal formula.

I was eager to visit this quite famous clinic with its storied past. Upon arriving at the Bio-Medical Center, Felipe dropped me off just outside the white two-story mansion, located in a quiet upscale neighborhood high on a hill, about ten minutes from the U.S. border. I had read that the mansion had been purchased at auction in the early 1960s, after the previous drug lord occupants had been sent to prison.

After entering through the tall metal gates attended by a guard, I walked along the path that hugged the circular driveway, past the giant round glass-and-screen aviary, en route to the reception area. I had been told that I would be meeting with and shadowing Robin, an American registered nurse who acts as clinic manager and patient liaison. I sat in the waiting area until Robin arrived. The morning was quiet and the atmosphere subdued as patients checked in and donned their long blue gowns to prepare for their initial exams. Later in the morning, however, the waiting room was bustling with conversation and gaiety, as strangers became friends. There were at least twenty patients at the clinic that day, and I was told that this was typical, that the clinic was always busy with patients from all over the country and, at times, the world.

After meeting with Robin and being introduced to the doctors and other staff, I mingled with the patients and their companions in the large waiting room with high ceilings and modest but comfortable furniture. The waiting room was adjacent to a beautiful tiled terrace that offered a wide view of Tijuana, with the Pacific Ocean, San Diego Bay, and the Tijuana hills beyond. I learned that some of the patients were at the clinic for the first time, while others were returning for follow-up visits.

I spent my two days at the Bio-Medical Center talking with patients and providing support to a few who were there on their own. I accompanied Robin as she checked in with all the patients, assessing their health status and making sure their needs were being met. Robin made sure that the patients who were in pain were seen first, and helped with any concerns the patients had in the course of the day.

Two women who I became acquainted with agreed to have me accompany them for their diagnostic tests and physician consultations. After one of the women had her blood drawn, I accompanied her to the little café in one wing of the clinic, where inexpensive breakfasts, fruit smoothies, and light lunches were served by kindly Mexican ladies. One of the kitchen ladies told me that she had worked there for about thirty years, and described how she loved seeing people returning and getting better. There was a menu with prices, but payment was on the honor system, with a self-pay box where people made their own change.

One of the patients I spent time with was Alicia, a cheerful and robust woman in her sixties who was returning to the clinic for what she hoped would be her final follow-up visit after being treated for breast cancer. Alicia told me that the clinic had gotten much busier after it was featured in the documentary *The Truth About Cancer*. She and her companion had driven through the night, and while he dozed in the chair next to her, Alicia told me the amazing story about how she originally ended up at the Bio-Medical Center—a story that most definitely included chance encounters, spiritual experiences, and answers to prayers.

A few years earlier, Alicia had made a big move across the country to settle in the town of her youth in the southwest, where she had planned to enjoy her retirement years while living closer to her daughter. Alicia hadn't lived in the small California desert town for twenty years, and was really excited to reconnect with her many old friends and acquaintances. She had barely finished unpacking when, one morning in the shower, she felt a small lump on her left breast. Alicia, a self-proclaimed optimist, didn't feel too alarmed, as she enjoyed excellent health and had barely even seen a doctor since she was a child. She made an appointment for a physical with the local family practice center and resumed settling into her new home.

Her doctor was not as blasé about the lump as Alicia was, and Alicia's alarm rose when he insisted she have a mammogram and ultrasound that same day. The findings of the tests were suggestive of cancer, and a biopsy was done shortly after. Alicia had breast cancer. She didn't want to tell anyone, as she needed time alone to process the bad news and decide what she should do. The night after getting the diagnosis, Alicia stayed up all night, crying and begging God to show her the way.

In the meantime, there was a confidentiality leak at one of the facilities where Alicia had received care, and old friends and acquaintances found out about Alicia's diagnosis. At the time, this was rather upsetting to her, but she later decided that it was a part of God's plan. That very first day after her diagnosis, nine old friends contacted Alicia to tell her how they had successfully been treated for a variety of cancers at the Bio-Medical Center. One of the friends had been treated twenty years previously, not long after Alicia had moved away, and the others had been successfully treated five or more years prior.

The success stories kept rolling in, and before the end of three days, Alicia had received thirty-five testimonials from acquaintances and friends of friends, all of whom had been treated at the Bio-Medical Center. One of the stories she heard was from a family member of a sixty-year-old man who had been so close to death that he had been carried to Bio-Medical by his family in a last-ditch effort to save his life. Alicia was told that the man recovered and had lived to be ninety years old. Alicia knew her prayers had been answered and that God was showing her the way.

At the end of the day, Alicia approached me to say good-bye. She cheerfully told me that her doctor did not find any signs of cancer and she did not need to take the Hoxsey tonic any longer.

I also briefly chatted with Kathy in the waiting room. She was from New Mexico, and her husband, Dennis, was returning for a follow-up visit for prostate cancer. Although we only talked for a short while, the story she told me is too ironic to omit. After her husband's doctor told the couple that Dennis had prostate cancer, and described the treatment regime, the doctor said to them, "Now don't you think of going off to Mexico for treatment." Kathy and Dennis didn't even know that treatment in Mexico was a possibility and were puzzled as to why the doctor would say such a thing.

The next day, while Kathy was out doing errands, she ran into an acquaintance and told her the bad news. Kathy was surprised to learn the woman's husband had also had prostate cancer, and that he had gone to the Bio-Medical Center in Tijuana for treatment and was doing fine years later. Needless to say, Kathy and Dennis did indeed go "off to Mexico for treatment."

I spoke with a few patients who did not have cancer. Some of the companions of patients were having complete physicals and lab work at costs far lower than in the United States. And one woman, accompanied by her husband and young children, had lupus, an autoimmune disease, and wished to avoid the immunosuppressive effects of conventional medical treatment.

I also met Julia and Bartek, an interesting European couple who were practicing naturopaths in Minneapolis. This was their first visit. Before his evaluation, Bartek told me that he had experienced some symptoms that were concerning and was worried he might have cancer, but he did not want to visit a conventional doctor. If it were cancer, he knew that he would not accept the chemotherapy, hormones, and/or radiation that would be advised. I saw them again later in the day, all smiles, and they told me it was not cancer.

I thoroughly enjoyed the time I spent at The Bio-Medical Center, and it is indeed a special place with a unique atmosphere. Although many people have achieved remission with the Hoxsey treatment, it does not help everyone. No treatment, conventional or alternative, has a 100% success rate. I am not sure that I would rely exclusively on the Hoxsey therapy if I were diagnosed with cancer, but I would certainly start the treatment promptly while I considered what other options to include in my recovery plan.

The Bio-Medical Center is the most affordable alternative cancer treatment option of those I visited in Tijuana. The cost is typically $1,000–3,000 for a new patient with cancer, and includes an exam and evaluation by a physician, diagnostic tests, and a three-month supply of the Hoxsey formula, along with other supplements. Most patients spend only one day at the clinic, where they meet with one of the doctors for an exam and a review of their past treatment and records, have any needed blood work and diagnostic tests, and are prescribed one of the Hoxsey herbal formulas. Other supplements are often prescribed, including Chinese herbs and an extract of yew.

Patients are given a packet that gives instructions for the prescribed herbal formulas and supplements, and outlines in detail the specific diet to be followed. Some people find the diet challenging to comply with, as it eliminates all tomato products, pork, refined flour, salt and sugar, and anything that contains vinegar, as these foods interfere with the actions of the Hoxsey herbal formula. Some patients receive intravenous therapies, such as laetrile and even low-dose chemotherapy, and stay longer than one day for treatment. The clinic has four rooms available at an additional cost to accommodate these patients. Many patients choose to stay at the Best Western Americana Inn in San Ysidro, California, just over the border, and take the provided medical van across the border early in the morning, returning that afternoon. Other patients stay at hotels closer to San Diego, and pay about $50 each way for a medical van to take them to the Bio-Medical Center and back.

There are many videos on YouTube about the Bio-Medical Center, and the documentary "The Quack Who Cured Cancer," about Harry Hoxsey and the political battles he fought, is also available on YouTube. There is an active Facebook page that contains many photos, videos, and patient testimonials, including offers by former patients welcoming others to contact them. For more information, visit http://www.hoxseybio-medical.com.

CHAPTER 8

A Bit of Tijuana Clinic History
The Oasis of Hope, Stella Maris,
Integrative Whole Health, and San Diego Clinics

For more than fifty years, Americans, Canadians, and people from all over the world have traveled to the many clinics of Tijuana to obtain treatments that are not available at home. The location of the clinics just over the border, less than twenty miles from San Diego, have made it relatively convenient for the thousands of Americans who seek alternative treatment. Many of the clinics established in the late 1960s and 1970s sprouted up as a result of one of the biggest American medical dramas of the twentieth century.

Laetrile, sometimes called vitamin B17, is a drug made from the natural compound amygdalin, found in the seeds of many fruits but commonly extracted from apricot pits. Although laetrile was known prior, it was in the 1960s that Ernst T. Krebs, Jr., began promoting laetrile as a promising treatment for cancer. In 1963, a book was published by Glenn Kittler entitled *Laetrile: Control for Cancer*, which became enormously popular, selling many thousands of copies.

Cancer patients began requesting laetrile, and several physicians in the United States provided it to their patients. There were research studies showing that laetrile was helpful to cancer patients, and many of the physicians using laetrile were providing evidence of its effectiveness in case reports. In his book *World Without Cancer: The Story of Vitamin B17*, first published in 1974, author G. Edward Griffin outlines the tumultuous history of laetrile and the medical and political forces that eventually led to it being discredited as a cancer therapy.

In the early 1970s, Kanematsu Sugiura, a distinguished senior Memorial Sloan Kettering scientist, conducted study after study that showed the effectiveness of laetrile on animals with malignant tumors. The drama around his research and the reaction of the Sloan Kettering administrators who covered up his positive results are chronicled in the 2014 film *Second Opinion: Laetrile at Sloan Kettering*, featuring Ralph Moss, then a science writer and assistant director of communications at Sloan Kettering who was fired for exposing the cover-up. Dr. Moss went on to become a tireless cancer treatment advocate, authoring books and articles that question conventional cancer treatment. When the FDA eventually made the interstate transport of laetrile illegal, and later made its administration illegal in the United States, people began traveling to Tijuana to receive it. In his article about the history of the Tijuana clinics, "Tijuana Cancer Clinics in the Post-Nafta Era,"[1] Dr. Moss reported data from a National Cancer Institute publication that stated that by 1978, about 70,000 American cancer patients had taken laetrile, and many of those had gone to Mexico to receive it.

The Mexican alternative cancer clinic phenomenon has, at its roots, strong influences from the United States and Germany. Much of the history of the Tijuana clinics begins not only with the story of Mildred Nelson and laetrile but with the stories of three other passionate, determined, and independent women. Charlotte Gerson and Ilise Issels, from Germany, and American Cecile Hoffman, all believed so strongly in cancer therapies that were suppressed in the United States that they opened, or inspired the opening of, treatment centers to provide them.

Cecile Hoffman was a married, upper-middle-class California school teacher when she was diagnosed with metastatic breast cancer in the early 1960s. After at least two surgeries and standard treatments, her doctors had no further hope to offer her. Cecile "gradually deteriorated so that she was in a lot of pain, even with drugs, and almost unable to walk. She was emaciated and unable to eat, and it appeared the end was approaching. She visited the local mortuary, picked out a coffin, laid down in it to see if it fit right, and prepared to have her remains shipped to the family burial plot in Michigan."[2]

Cecile's husband happened across Glen Kittler's book about laetrile, and with renewed hope, Cecile was determined to find a doctor who would administer it to her. Cecile was unable to find an American doctor who would do so, but she located physician Ernesto Contreras, a former Mexican army pathologist practicing medicine in Tijuana, who was willing. According to historical accounts, Cecile improved with the laetrile treatments, and by March of 1964, her X-rays revealed that the tumors had disappeared. Cecile went on to promote alternative cancer therapies and eventually co-founded the organization Cancer Victims and Friends, which had its first convention in 1965 and eventually became the Cancer Control Society, still active today. Ernesto Contreras went on to establish the largest laetrile clinic in the world— the Del Mar Medical Center and Hospital—which eventually became the **Oasis of Hope** hospital, now a thriving full-service integrative cancer hospital in Playas, operated by Ernesto Contreras's son, physician Francisco Contreras, and his grandson, Daniel Kennedy.

I was very eager to visit the Oasis of Hope and contacted the hospital when I was arranging my own tour of the clinics, but I was rather curtly told that visits are not allowed. I passed the hospital every day, walking from the Dali Suites hotel to the beach, and, on occasion, I stepped into the very pretty garden courtyard entryway to the four-story, glass-faced modern building that housed the Oasis of Hope. I also frequently greeted people who appeared to be Americans, often sitting on the curb, smoking, as I passed by.

On a later trip to Tijuana I was able to visit the Oasis of Hope on the Cancer Control Society bus tour of four clinics. The tour the society offers after their annual convention on Labor Day weekend is very popular, and we were a large group as we filed off the bus. On this tour I became friendly with Joy, a woman who had recently been diagnosed with cancer, and in addition to taking the tour, she had scheduled private visits to additional clinics not included on the tour. The people on the bus were an interesting mix. Some of them had cancer, including a man from Australia, and were exploring treatment options. Others were health professionals who had an interest in alternative cancer treatment. One woman had lost her husband to cancer after a long illness, and she was creating a documentary about alternative cancer treatment options. One of the administrators of the Cancer Tutor website joined us, as well as a man from Washington, D.C., who provides information to people who are interested in alternative cancer treatment. Another woman on the tour had been treated conventionally for breast cancer in the past, but she wanted to learn about alternative treatment options should she experience a recurrence.

Our large group was escorted through the courtyard and reception area of the Oasis of Hope into a ballroom-sized dining room. In anticipation of our arrival, numerous round tables were set with white tablecloths for lunch and presentations by the staff. Daniel Kennedy gave an overview of the treatment philosophy and the history of the Oasis of Hope, and the director of oncology programs, physician Francisco Cecena, fielded our questions about cancer treatment. Lunch was vegan, delicious and elegantly presented.

Small groups of five or six were invited to tour the cancer treatment unit with English-speaking staff escorts, and we were shown an unoccupied patient room that was large and clean, with basic furnishings and included a small terrace with views toward the sea. The rooms were arranged around a central nurse's station, and I chatted a bit with one of the nurses. We were shown the small chapel and adjacent private garden courtyard. I appreciated the way the privacy of the patients was protected during a visit by such a large group as ours, and I presumed that the patients were in the treatment rooms or common areas that we were not shown.

The Oasis of Hope and medical director Dr. Francisco Contreras are very well known globally. Dr. Contreras is an oncologist, having done post-medical school studies in Vienna. He frequently presents at numerous conferences, and many of his interviews and presentations can be found on YouTube. The Oasis of Hope employs an experienced team of physicians, many of whom have worked at the facility for a number of years.

The model of cancer treatment is called Contreras Alternative Cancer Treatment, and it integrates conventional cancer treatments, including low-dose chemotherapy and radiation therapy, with numerous alternative therapies, including hyperthermia, laetrile, dendritic cell vaccines, and others.

The Oasis of Hope states that its treatment programs result in a survival rate that is three times higher than the U.S. national average. Cancer nutrition is a major focus, with a plant-based, mostly vegan, low-sugar diet provided. Nutritional education and cooking classes are included in the treatment program.

Patients are encouraged to bring a companion, whose room and board is included in the basic price. The cost of treatment at Oasis of Hope can be quite high, depending on length of stay and the type of treatments required. One of the criticisms I have often heard is that the costs can rise far beyond that which is initially quoted, as various treatments and interventions are gradually added to a patient's treatment plan. For more information, visit http://www.oasisofhope.com.

I visited other clinics whose medical directors trace their lineage back to the laetrile boon era. Some of them worked with Dr. Ernesto Contreras, of the Oasis of Hope, before his death in 2003, while others worked at the Manner Clinic; some worked at both clinics.

The Manner Clinic, founded by American scientist Harold Manner, left a lasting legacy on the Tijuana cancer clinic scene. A Loyola University biologist who had originally dedicated himself to the study of the developmental biology of fish and animals, Manner became interested in the use of laetrile, enzymes, and other substances to treat cancer. He established the Metabolic Research Foundation in Illinois to promote his Metabolic Therapy for the treatment of cancer. However, Manner was subject to the same FDA harassment as other doctors and scientists who went against the grain of mainstream medicine, and in 1982 the foundation took over the Cydel Clinic, one of the early Tijuana laetrile clinics that sprouted up in the 1970s as laetrile became outlawed in the United States.

Manner renamed Cydel the Manner Clinic, making the Manner Metabolic Therapy available to American cancer patients. Manner's metabolic therapy included many therapies that are offered in the Tijuana clinics today, including the Manner Cocktail, a combination of laetrile, enzymes, vitamins, and dimethyl sulfoxide (DMSO). Although Manner died in 1988, the Manner Clinic remained open until the early 1990s and several of the former Manner Clinic doctors later opened their own clinics after beginning their careers with Manner.

✒

Dr. Gilberto Alvarez, of the **Stella Maris Clinic**, is one such physician who, after working for four years with Dr. Ernesto Contreras, (the first doctor to open his doors to Cecile Hoffman and other Americans seeking laetrile), became the medical director of the Manner Clinic. Dr. Alvarez remained at the Manner Clinic for ten years before opening Stella Maris in 1993.

Dr. Alvarez is well known for his expertise, experience, and friendly, kind nature, and when I called him, he did not hesitate to invite me to visit the following day. I had a bit of an adventure finding the clinic and discovered, not for the first time, that street numbers do not always follow a consecutive and logical pattern in Tijuana. I had taken an Uber to the area where I thought the clinic was and looked for quite some time before asking a young man for directions. He hailed a cab for me to help me find the building a mile or two further down the busy boulevard.

I found the Stella Maris Clinic to be a sparkling, bright, and modern space, located on the second floor of a professional office complex. When I entered the Stella Maris suite, I felt as if I could have easily been in any modern medical office in the United States. I was greeted by Dr. Alvarez's nurse, Ofelia, who has worked with him for over twenty years, and Dr. Alvarez's wife, Linda, who speaks fluent, accent-free English and serves as clinic manager and patient advocate. After only a few minutes' wait, Dr. Alvarez greeted me and took me to his office, which was separated from the intravenous therapy treatment room by only a transparent wall. The intravenous therapy room was a bright and comfortable space with a wall-to-wall window and several large reclining chairs.

Dr. Alvarez showed me around the treatment area behind his office where hyperthermia and other therapies are administered, and explained the various equipment he uses. I noticed that the walls of the room were plastered with the many certificates that he has received from participating in educational programs and conferences around the globe, including those for studies in hyperthermia, enzyme therapy, and other therapies for cancer. Also displayed was a certificate showing that Dr. Alvarez had passed the United States medical boards, and Dr. Alvarez told me he is eligible to apply for licensure in the United States if he chooses to do so.

I found Dr. Alvarez to be a very kind, humble, and soft-spoken man, and I wished that I had made a list of very specific questions, as he was rather quiet and not inclined to make any attempts to "sell" his treatment program. His depth and breadth of experience was apparent as he described a few of the cases he has treated successfully over the years. He told me that many of his patients are referred to him by former patients, and on the day of my visit, one of his patients was a man who knew someone who had been treated for brain cancer by Dr. Alvarez many years ago, who was alive and doing well. It was clear to me that Dr. Alvarez is a most attentive and compassionate physician who is very visible and accessible to his patients. He had just returned from vacation, and rather than entrust the care of his patients to other doctors, he had closed the clinic.

Dr. Alvarez performs an individualized assessment of every patient, and treatment protocols are highly individualized. A large variety of therapies are available, including hyperthermia, immunotherapies, laetrile/vitamin C infusions, and many others. The Stella Maris Clinic is an outpatient clinic that offers these individualized treatment programs five days per week, typically for three weeks per visit. Patients receive a discount at one of the many nearby hotels, and the Stella Maris staff provides a healthy breakfast and lunch to patients on each treatment day. The cost varies according to the needs of each patient, and ranges about $6,000–7,000 per week. The Stella Maris website, http://www.stellamarisclinic.com, is very educational, with in-depth descriptions of all the various components of treatment.

∽

Dr. Jose Henriquez, medical director of the **Integrative Whole Health Clinic**, is another highly experienced physician in Tijuana who obtained his early experience treating cancer as an intern at the original Del Mar Hospital (now Oasis of Hope) with Ernesto Contreras. Dr. Henriquez was also an attending physician at the Manner Clinic, and later at the International Bio-Care Hospital, before establishing the Integrative Whole Health Clinic in 2009. I contacted Dr. Henriquez prior to arriving in Tijuana, and he responded to my inquiry with a warm welcome to visit him and his clinic.

Dr. Henriquez met me at his Zona Rio office before driving me to his small inpatient clinic in a private villa, about ten minutes away. The clinic was located in a quiet and beautiful suburban setting that had the ambiance of a new upscale San Diego neighborhood. Dr. Henriquez was welcoming, professional, and informative, and as he had completed an undergraduate degree in the United States, his English was perfect, with barely an accent as he answered my many questions.

When we met, Dr. Henriquez had just returned from Riga, Latvia, where he had completed the physician credentialing program that would allow him to administer Rigvir, a promising new oncolytic viral therapy for cancer which is approved by the governments of Latvia and Georgia. In addition to attending educational programs in Europe, Dr. Henriquez teaches principles of integrative cancer treatment in Asia, and is highly credentialed and experienced in the use of hyperthermia.

I found the two-story villa that houses the clinic elegant and beautifully furnished, with a spacious living area and numerous treatment rooms in addition to the patient rooms. I appreciated the private, home-like environment of this clinic, combined with an intensive individualized treatment program, and sensed I would feel very comfortable and safe receiving treatment there. I learned that the clinic treats only four patients at a given time to ensure the patients receive personalized attention and treatment. The clinic, I was told, is staffed with nurses around the clock, and I met Dr. Maria del Refugio Garcia Moreno, a very kind and engaging young doctor who assists Dr. Henriquez and joined us for the tour and discussions during my visit.

I met three patients who were receiving treatment, and their companions, and all expressed positive feelings about their care. Like many of the inpatient facilities I visited, a companion is welcome to share the patient's room, and their room and board is included in the cost of treatment. The diet is mostly organic and vegetarian, and modified according to patient needs. A very sweet lady who managed the modern and spotless kitchen served me green juice as Dr. Henriquez, Dr. Moreno, and I sat in the dining room that faced the courtyard patio and discussed the treatment protocols of the clinic.

Dr. Henriquez said that most of his patients are Stage IV cancer patients who have received conventional treatment, and have not been given any hope by conventional oncology. He said about 75% of his patients go into remission after his treatment, or have a vastly improved quality of life. Dr. Henriquez expressed his strong belief that if a comprehensive treatment program such as his could be included in a clinical trial, the results would be far superior to the results of standard conventional treatments. Dr. Henriquez also gave me a tutorial about the genetic issues related to cancer, and although I tried to keep up, it was a bit over my head. It was obvious, though, that I was speaking with a doctor who was extremely knowledgeable and experienced in the treatment of cancer. He also expressed enthusiasm about live cell therapy, a commonly used therapy in Europe that increases the strength of the immune system and strengthens organs. After the tour and very educational conversation, I was treated to a brief tour of some of Tijuana, as Dr. Henriquez kindly drove me back to my hotel in Playas, continuing the discussion of many issues related to cancer treatment.

The Integrative Whole Health Clinic offers a variety of therapies based on an individual assessment of each patient's health status. These include hyperthermia, intravenous therapies including laetrile and vitamin C, various supplements for immune stimulation, and oxygen therapies. Dendritic cell vaccines and other immunotherapies are also provided. Detoxification therapy is provided in the form of coffee and flax enemas, dietary interventions, and use of a spa system that provides heat therapy and lymphatic massage. Dr. Henriquez is experienced with low-dose chemotherapy with insulin potentiation therapy (IPT) and/or hyperthermia, and it is available to those who request it. The cost for four weeks of treatment was under $30,000 in 2016 and included a six-month supply of dendritic cell vaccines to be administered at home. I found this cost to be quite reasonable compared to many of the other inpatient clinics, considering the personalized attention by a highly experienced physician, elegant home-like atmosphere, the therapies offered, and four-week length of treatment. For more information, visit the clinic's website at http://www.iwhc.com.

One of my favorite and longest clinic visits was to the **San Diego Clinic**, operated by Dr. Filiberto Muñoz, a well-known and respected doctor who has been treating people with cancer for decades. Dr. Muñoz is another physician who obtained his early experience treating cancer with Dr. Ernesto Contreras, as well as during shorter periods of employment at the Manner Clinic and the Bio-Medical Center. Dr. Muñoz said that he and Mildred Nelson remained very good friends, even though he left the Bio-Medical Center because of his desire to incorporate other therapies and opened the San Diego Clinic in 1997.

I had heard many wonderful things about Dr. Muñoz prior to meeting him and so I had especially looked forward to this visit. Before going to Tijuana, I became acquainted with Claudia, a woman in her seventies who had been treated for invasive breast cancer several years prior by him. Claudia had nothing but positive feelings toward Dr. Muñoz, and she was the person who first told me about the elastogram technology for breast cancer screening. She and her husband, who was also treated successfully for oral cancer by Dr. Muñoz, continue to make the trip from the Los Angeles area at least twice a year for follow-up visits.

At the Dali Suites hotel, I had met Camille and Phil, an older British couple who had made several visits from England for the treatment of Phil's prostate cancer that had metastasized to the bone. Camille, a tiny gray-haired lady in her seventies, told me that Phil's bone lesions were now gone and that they were very happy with Dr. Muñoz and the treatment. One day I had a conversation with Camille about the differences between the American and British health care systems and why she and Phil had decided to come to Mexico for treatment. In her strong British accent, and with a twinkle in her eye, Camille said, "Yes, you Americans must pay to be killed with chemo. In Britain, it is free."

A young Canadian couple, Lily and Sean, were also staying at the Dali Suites for treatment of Lily's rare cancer. Sean told me that they had been referred to Dr. Muñoz by Burton Goldberg, a well-known integrative cancer treatment advocate and author of *Alternative Medicine: The Definitive Guide*, after Canadian oncologists did not have any promising treatment options to offer her. Sean said that many of Dr. Muñoz's patients are referred by Goldberg, and when I looked at Goldberg's website, still present after his recent death at age 90, I saw many positive testimonials from patients who had received treatment from Dr. Muñoz. Dr. Muñoz is also mentioned in Suzanne Somers' book, *KNOCKOUT: Interviews with Doctors Who Are Curing Cancer—And How to Prevent Getting It in the First Place.*

Despite its name, the San Diego Clinic is located in Tijuana's Zona Rio District. It is an outpatient clinic within walking distance of the California border. I took an Uber from Playas to Zona Rio, as Uber had proved a reliable and less expensive option than a taxi, although none of the drivers seemed to speak English. I had a morning appointment to meet with Dr. Muñoz, and an afternoon appointment with the radiologist who was to perform a breast ultrasound with elastography exam on me. After the Uber driver dropped me off, I once again had trouble finding the exact building. I eventually found the clinic with the assistance of a very kind parking lot attendant who works for the San Diego Clinic, and who walked me into the building himself.

After checking in at the front desk, I sat in the spartan but spacious waiting area that contained a small café with about six tables in one corner of the room. Dr. Muñoz greeted me warmly and led me to his office, where he talked with me for over an hour. I was immediately put at ease by his friendly, down-to-earth demeanor, and I found him to be an extremely authentic man whose integrity, honesty, and dedication to helping people came through very strongly throughout our time together.

Dr. Muñoz shared his passion for immunotherapies, and described the different types that he uses at the clinic. He was very enthused about a type of immunotherapy called "tumor-infiltrating lymphocyte vaccine," which he described as very effective when he can secure a tumor sample with which to make the vaccine. He showed me a thick textbook on his desk written by American physician and scientist Stephen A. Rosenberg, called *Principles and Practice of the Biological Therapy of Cancer.* With a degree of exasperation in his voice, he said that the Americans [oncologists] know this information but they just don't use it. He also expressed his frustration that most of the immunotherapy clinical trials are done after a patient has sustained immune system damage from chemotherapy, when in fact the immune system needs to be functioning as well as possible for immunotherapies to work. He said he does all of his continuing education through programs and physicians in Germany, and on his computer screen he showed me a German online immunotherapy course he was currently attending.

Dr. Munoz spoke passionately about the epidemic of cancer in the United States, and expressed his frustration that more was not being done to educate people about cancer prevention. He told me that he offers a complete evaluation of cancer risk for people without known cancer for $500. Among other tests, this evaluation includes the ENOX-2 protein blood test that can detect cancer years before it can be diagnosed with conventional screening methods. This is a simplified version of the Oncoblot blood test that had, until mid-2016, been available in the United States through integrative practitioners and cost about $1,000. (At the time of this writing, the Oncoblot has not been available for many months due to a change in ownership of the company, but the Oncoblot website states that the test will be available in the future.) Whereas the Oncoblot can discern the exact organ creating the high level of the cancer protein, the ENOX-2 test reports only a numeric value that indicates the concern for a developing cancer. Dr. Muñoz told me that a score of under 30 is considered negative, while for a score of 30–100, an oral supplement called Capsol-T (a high-potency blend of green tea and capsicum red pepper that has some published evidence for lowering ENOX-2 protein) is recommended. Treatment is advised for a score of over 100.

I asked Dr. Muñoz if he was seeing an increase in the number of patients who had tried to treat their own cancer, and he said that he had. He said that patients often come to see him for an initial consultation, with piles of supplements they have been taking, reacting to every media report about the latest and greatest natural product to cure cancer. When he performs individualized testing to assess what supplements each patient needs, he often finds that most of what the person has been taking is not needed or helpful.

Dr. Munoz told me more than once that he did not want to waste people's money, and would not accept patients he did not think he could help. He said he uses the RGCC blood test (Greece Test) to determine what natural substances an individual's cancer is sensitive to, pointing out that therapies such as intravenous vitamin C have become expensive, and not all cancer responds to it.

Dr. Munoz stressed that his protocols are very individualized, and that his method includes changing approaches and adjusting treatments over time because treatments that were once helpful can stop being effective. Dr. Munoz said that he will only treat ten patients at one time, and has no interest in expanding, as he wants to be able to personally provide the most individualized treatment. When I asked Dr. Muñoz about a typical length of treatment for his patients, I found that he is uncompromising about this and said that the worst thing you can do is treat cancer for a little while and then stop treatment. For those with advanced cancer, he said he typically treats his patients six days a week for at least six weeks, and after a few weeks at home, with home treatments, they return for another round of treatment for a few more weeks. He said that his patients continue seeing him for some length of time, depending on their progress.

I asked Dr. Muñoz about the type of diet he recommends to his patients. He said he does not prescribe a rigid diet and that one of the physicians at the clinic who has specialized cancer nutrition training meets with each patient. She helps them add beneficial foods and remove detrimental nutritional choices such as processed foods, excessive sugar, and animal protein while honoring their culture and native diet. He said he thinks this approach works best to improve compliance with making the dietary changes that support recovery.

When I asked Dr. Muñoz how he responds when potential patients ask him about his success rates, he said he can put 50% of advanced cancer patients into remission, where they are able to resume normal lives, and helps others by improving their quality of life. He does not accept patients whom he feels he cannot help because he does not want them to spend their money unnecessarily. He also said that he does not accept patients with brain cancer or leukemia, but instead refers brain cancer patients to Dr. Stanislaw Burzynski, in Houston, saying he has the best results of anyone in the world.

During our conversation about the ENOX-2 protein test, I decided to have the test while there, at the clinic. I assumed my only option was to pay the $500 for the evaluation that included the test, and I was prepared to spend the money, but Dr. Muñoz said I could have just that one blood test alone, at a cost of only $150. He walked me down one of the two corridors that had offices and treatment rooms to the large intravenous therapy room and nurses station. I sat in one of the comfy reclining chairs in the plain but clean room, along with several patients who were connected to intravenous drips, and one of the nurses came and effortlessly drew my blood. I was told it would take about two weeks to receive my results, which would be emailed to me. I learned a great deal during my time with Dr. Muñoz, and wished that I had recorded all the information he shared. He most definitely lived up to all the praise that I had heard prior to meeting him.

I went back to the front reception area as I still had an hour before my appointment for the breast exam, and sat in the little café to have a snack. I was joined by a man who had accompanied his adult son for treatment of an advanced cancer. Bill told me that he and his son had visited a few Tijuana clinics, including one of the larger multi-physician hospitals. After reviewing his son's records, a doctor at one of these hospitals, (Bill would not tell me which hospital) advised Bill to take his son to Dr. Muñoz, due to his expertise with his son's particular case of a complicated cancer.

I soon met the radiologist and had the exam, before catching a ride along with Lily and Sean back to Playas with one of the employees of the clinic. Many, but not all of Dr. Muñoz's patients stay at the Dali Suites, and transportation is provided to and from Playas and the Dali Suites daily.

The San Diego Clinic provides outpatient treatment six days per week. Numerous therapies are employed based on continual assessment of progress and cancer response. These comprise various immunotherapies, including the prostate-specific immunotherapy called Prostvac, which is not yet available in the U.S. outside of clinical trials. The clinic offers hyperthermia and low-dose chemotherapy with insulin potentiation therapy (IPT) or hyperthermia, intravenous therapies of natural substances, and conventional medications, as indicated. Dr. Muñoz is *assisted by other physicians, but he determines the plan of care and supervises the treatment of all patients. Costs are relatively reasonable at the San Diego Clinic and credit cards are accepted. I was told that the cost ranges from $4,000–5,000 a week for most people, but for some with more specialized needs the price can go up to $6,000 a week. Certain medications and supplements are not included in the basic price. For more information, visit http://www.sdiegoclinic.com.*

(As a postscript, I received the results of the ENOX-2 blood test after I returned home, and was dismayed to find I had a borderline result in the 30s. I decided to make some lifestyle tweaks and have the Oncoblot done when it is available again, or to return to the San Diego Clinic in one year to repeat the test before starting treatment with Capsol-T. From my research about Capsol-T, it is rather expensive and does not work for everyone. Months after I received the results of my blood test, I spoke with a woman whose husband, a physician himself, was treated at the San Diego Clinic for confirmed Stage IV prostate cancer. She told me that her husband's ENOX-2 blood test was also in the 30s, despite having active cancer, so it is clearly not a 100% accurate test. As I mentioned earlier, my breast ultrasound with thermography was completely normal, and I was given the CD of the exam to show my doctor.)

CHAPTER 9
A Trip Down the Pacific Coast
Baja Health and Wellness, CHIPSA, St. Andrews, Northern Baja Healing Center, and Sanoviv Medical Institute

Recalling the previous discussion of the Gerson Therapy, and that of the four passionate and influential women in the history of cancer treatment in Tijuana, perhaps the best known is Charlotte Gerson, who was responsible for bringing her late father's cancer therapy to Mexico so it could be made available to patients outside the reach of the American medical authorities. Charlotte Gerson has been a very animated, articulate, and passionate alternative cancer treatment advocate for decades, and has been featured in numerous films and interviews. She remained very active with the Gerson Institute until in her early nineties, when a series of falls and fractures slowed her down. Her last interview at age ninety-three demonstrated her mental sharpness and continued dedication to the Gerson Therapy, as she spoke about using the Gerson nutritional principles to help heal her injuries.

Charlotte was just a teenager in 1936 when her father moved from Germany to the United States, but she was very involved in her father's work, learned the therapy, and witnessed the cures that the Gerson Therapy produced. Dr. Gerson's therapies and theories lay dormant after his death in 1959, until Norman Fritz, an engineer with a great interest in alternative cancer treatment who had been involved with the Cancer Control Society, contacted Charlotte Gerson in 1974, suggesting they work together to reestablish the Gerson Therapy. Charlotte, with the help of Norman Fritz and doctors in Mexico, established the first Gerson clinic in an old resort hotel on the Pacific coast, near Tijuana, in 1977, and named it the Hospital de la Gloria. When the clinic burned down, Charlotte established a new Gerson Institute clinic in Playas. It offers only the original Gerson Therapy. I was told that the clinic does not accept visitors, so I did not have the opportunity to visit.

Another German influence on the Tijuana cancer clinic phenomenon occurred in the late 1980s, when Josef Issels, MD, and his wife, Ilse Marie, arrived in Southern California with the immunotherapy protocols he had been using to treat cancer in Germany since 1951. In Germany, Dr. Issels had established the first hospital in the world dedicated to integrative cancer treatment, which included various immunotherapies, nutrition, and hyperthermia. The hospital grew to 120 beds and had a research department dedicated to the study and development of cancer vaccines. Dr. Issels became well known in Germany for improved outcomes in treating patients who were considered terminal. After he retired in 1987, he and his wife, Ilse Marie, settled in California and introduced what is now called the "Issels Integrative Immuno-Oncology" treatment model to Mexico.

According to Dan Rogers, MD, one of the early physicians who worked with Charlotte Gerson and who has been treating cancer patients in Mexico for over thirty years, Dr. Issels contacted him before he and Ilse Marie came to California. Dr. Rogers told me that Issels had met Gerson in Germany at some point and wanted to integrate Gerson's nutritional therapy with Issels' immunotherapy, convinced that the combined outcome would be better than either alone. At that time, Dr. Rogers was working at CHIPSA hospital, (Centro Hospitalario Internacional del Pacifico), and for about three years Issels worked with Dr. Rogers and the other medical staff, teaching them the procedures for creating and administering autologous vaccines.

Dr. Issels died in 1997 at age ninety, and a tribute to him in the *Journal of Alternative and Complementary Medicine* called him "The Father of Integrative Medicine." Many of the doctors treating cancer in Tijuana were introduced to his work, either directly or indirectly, sparking the inclusion of immunotherapies in cancer treatment in Tijuana long before the United States' FDA approved the first immunotherapy cancer vaccine.

After Dr. Issels' death, Ilse Marie became the fourth passionate and independent woman who played a role in influencing cancer treatment in Mexico when she established an Issels Immunotherapy program at the Oasis of Hope Hospital with their son, Christian, a doctor of naturopathy. Later, Ilse Marie and Christian opened their own treatment center in the large and modern Angeles Hospital in Tijuana's Zona Rio, where it remains today. This Issels Immunotherapy Inpatient Center also has an outpatient clinic in Santa Barbara, California, where patients typically receive treatment deemed legal in the United States before going to the inpatient Issels program in Tijuana for the immunotherapies and other treatments that are not FDA approved. I did not have the opportunity to visit the Issels Center, but I was able to visit other clinics that combine the therapies of Gerson and Issels with other treatments.

∽

One of these clinics that I visited, the **Baja Health and Wellness Center**, offers "Gerson Plus Therapy" and is operated by Dan Rogers, MD, in Playas. Dr. Rogers is an American who completed undergraduate degrees in the U.S. but went to medical school in Mexico. He completed a family practice residency in the U.S. after medical school, but chose to return to Mexico in 1978 to work with Charlotte Gerson at the first Gerson Center. In the 1980s Dr. Rogers became chief of staff at CHIPSA, incorporating the Issels vaccines and other therapies with the Gerson Therapy. He eventually went into solo practice and established his own clinic. Dr. Rogers welcomed a visit on short notice, and I gratefully accepted his offer to pick me up at the Dali Suites, sparing me the long walk and adventure of finding my way.

The attractive and spacious villa that housed the Baja Health and Wellness Center was located in a very pleasant and peaceful neighborhood, a distance from the bustling and noisy commercial center of Playas. I particularly liked the large rooftop sun terrace that had views of the Pacific just a few blocks away. The clinic was clean, comfortable, and simply furnished, with the patient rooms on the upper floors. The ground level housed the kitchen, where the classic Gerson diet and juices are prepared, and a treatment area with a variety of medical equipment.

Dr. Rogers told me that most of his patients are between fifty and seventy years old, have Stage IV cancer, and have been sent home to die by conventional oncology. He said that he can save about half of his patients, and described brief case histories of a few of these successes. Dr. Rogers also told me about some of his patients who did not have cancer but were treated for mental illnesses and other conditions. He said that he has found that even those with mental illnesses benefit from the support of the various immunotherapies he offers.

I found Dr. Rogers to be very professional, passionate, and knowledgeable about all aspects of A/I (alternative/integrative) cancer treatment. I was interested to learn about all the paperwork and costs that are necessary to legally operate a clinic in Mexico. Dr. Rogers said that every therapy must be individually approved and registered with the government, with each application for a specific therapy requiring a fee. With his extensive experience of treating cancer, Dr. Rogers has been active in educating others about the Gerson Therapy and other alternative approaches to cancer treatment, and there are many videos of Dr. Rogers' presentations on YouTube.

Dr. Rogers offers the classic Gerson Therapy, Coley's fluids, intravenous therapies including laetrile and vitamin C, immersion hyperthermia, autologous vaccines, and many other supplements and therapies based on an individualized treatment plan. The clinic serves only five patients at a given time, who receive personalized attention and treatment. A three-week individualized course of treatment including the complete Gerson Therapy, all of the additional therapies, and a six-month supply of immunotherapy vaccines to administer at home costs $49,000, including room and board for a companion and transportation from the San Diego airport. The clinic also offers the classic Gerson Therapy as a stand-alone treatment, at the cost of $5,000 per week. For more information, visit http://www.gersonplus.com.

∾

Later, I had an appointment to visit **CHIPSA Hospital**, a well-known and long-established cancer treatment hospital that integrates the Gerson Therapy with immunotherapies and other A/I therapies. I spoke with their patient representative on three occasions and had submitted my R.N. license and letter of introduction. Yet, when I arrived at my appointed time in the lobby of the five-story building in the busy commercial district of Playas, I was not permitted to visit the hospital or speak with the doctors.

The American patient representative was happy to try to answer my questions in his spartan ground floor office, but I was apologetically told that the doctors were very busy and were not comfortable with me visiting the clinic area. He told me that the hospital had been recently purchased by an American businessman and spoke about CHIPSA's plans to renovate and create a hospital that maintained the same high standards as American hospitals. Since this is where Bailey O'Brien had received successful treatment for Stage IV melanoma, and I had heard of many other success stories from patients treated at CHIPSA, I was disappointed that I was not permitted to visit the clinic area or meet any of the staff.

Joy, my acquaintance from the Cancer Control Society tour of clinics who was considering treatment for herself, had arranged a private visit to CHIPSA, as it was not included on the bus tour. Joy said the staff had been very warm and friendly and that she had been very impressed with the kindness and experience of Dr. Lopez, the doctor she had met with. Joy wondered if I had not been allowed to visit due to the clean but somewhat shabby and bare-boned nature of the physical environment, and she, too, had been told of their renovation efforts and plans.

CHIPSA offers a modified version of the Gerson Therapy, including the basic diet, frequent vegetable juices, supplements, and coffee enemas. Many other therapies are combined with the Gerson Therapy, prescribed by one of the many physicians on staff at CHIPSA. Coley's toxins and dendritic-cell and other immunotherapy vaccines are an integral part of the protocols, as well as hyperthermia, laetrile and vitamin C infusions, and various supplements. Low-dose chemotherapy with IPT (insulin potentiation therapy) is prescribed for some patients. CHIPSA's medical staff includes doctors with many years of experience treating cancer, as well as some with specialized post-medical school training.

The hospital has its own pharmacy, laboratory, X-ray, and ultrasound *facilities, as well as the capacity to treat very ill patients and perform surgeries. Companions are welcomed and encouraged, and each room contains two beds to accommodate the patient plus their companion. I was not able to obtain specific cost information for CHIPSA, but the patient advocate did not disagree with my guess of a range of $30,000–40,000 for a three-week course of treatment. In addition to an informative website, CHIPSA has an active Facebook page that features many patient testimonials, information about the therapies, and various updates. A 2017 update states that CHIPSA has hired a former M.D. Anderson Cancer Center oncologist as their director of oncology research, and also lists Gar Hildenbrand as their director of epidemiology. Since my visit, CHIPSA has also begun offering outpatient treatment.*

Although I continue to hear positive comments regarding the caring demeanor of the doctors and patient care staff, several reports from patients who have received treatment since the change in management have contained complaints about the practices and ethics of the business office and administration. These patients advise careful review of an itemized treatment contract, including the costs of potential discharge medications. They also advise providing payment in weekly installments. For more information, visit http://www.chipsahospital.org.

On another day, I had planned to visit **St. Andrews**, a small outpatient clinic where Gar Hildenbrand, the Gerson consultant who had worked with Bailey O'Brien at CHIPSA, was serving in the consultant role. I had become friends with Grace, a woman from New York who was being treated for breast cancer at St. Andrews and was staying at the Dali Suites hotel, and I was looking forward to seeing her and meeting Gar who, with his wife, Christeene, has been involved with alternative cancer treatment in Mexico for decades.

Grace and other patients of St. Andrews who were staying at the Dali Suites told me it was only a ten-minute walk, so I set out on a hot afternoon for my scheduled visit. I walked and walked the streets of Playas for over an hour, unable to find the clinic. The address I was given apparently did not exist, and residents of the area where the street number should have been had never heard of a clinic in their residential neighborhood.

Finally, I asked a man outside a local business for help, and he spoke rapidly to his sister in Spanish. The only words I understood were those about him giving her money for gas. The woman spoke to me in English, suggesting I hop in her car and we would find this clinic. I was hot and tired at this point, so I got in the car, grateful for the help and rest. When I started speaking Spanish with Silvia, she insisted, "No, we speak in English. I want to practice."

Silvia and I drove all over Playas, and, curiously, before I had even told Silvia about my project and that I was a nurse, she told me all about her and her husband's autoimmune illnesses and asked me if I knew anything about the natural supplement she was taking. I had not heard of the supplement, but I looked it up on my phone as Silvia drove and saw that it was indeed quite popular. We then had a conversation about the role of nutrition for health and I learned about the challenges of eating a healthy diet in Mexico, where meat and refined foods are popular and abundant, and fresh vegetables are expensive.

We never found the clinic, but I made a new friend, and Silvia ended up dropping me off at the Walmart where Gar and Grace eventually came to pick me up to take me to the clinic. Most of the staff had gone home by the time I arrived, so I did not get the opportunity to meet with the doctors. I was able to take a quick tour of the clinic, which appeared to be a private home in a quiet residential area. It was clean, comfortable, and very simply furnished. It turned out that the doctor at St. Andrews had given Gar the right street name but the wrong house number, and I am still unsure whether this was an innocent mistake or not, as the address given on the St. Andrews website was also incorrect.

I met a few patients of St. Andrews at the Dali Suites and have stayed in touch with them. Unfortunately, for a variety of reasons, they do not recommend this clinic, despite their high regard for Gar and the therapies offered. The association with the Gerson Research Organization, the relatively reasonable cost of about $5,000 per week, and the availability of Coley's toxins and the other therapies are what contributed to these people's choice of this clinic. In addition, the medical *director is a highly qualified, board certified oncological surgeon.*

The clinic offers a six-day-per-week outpatient treatment program with a modified Gerson Therapy, Coley's toxins, immersion hyperthermia, chelation, and various intravenous therapies and supplements. Low-dose chemotherapy with IPT is also part of the treatment for some patients. At the time of my visit, Gar and Christeene spent two days each week at the clinic, facilitating the Gerson Therapy and other components of the treatment and assisting patients with a variety of needs and requests. Length of treatment is at least three weeks. For more information, visit http://www.standrewsclinic.com.

After the visit to the clinic, Gar, Christeene, Grace, and I went to one of the most popular restaurants in Playas, El Yogurt Place. I found Gar and Christeene to be very fascinating people, and they treated me to an extensive history lesson about how they became involved with alternative cancer treatment, the Gerson Therapy, Charlotte Gerson, Coley's toxins, and related subjects. Gar was a southern California playwright, and Christeene a professional opera singer, before they became involved in cancer treatment. Gar had heard about Max Gerson and was interested in writing a play about him. When Gar asked Charlotte Gerson for her help, she told Gar that she was far too busy with the clinic in Mexico to spend any time with him. Gar offered to help her and became fascinated and impressed with the Gerson Therapy and Dr. Gerson's writings and case studies. Gar also discovered that the Gerson Therapy greatly improved some health issues he had been struggling with. Gar took a deep dive into the world of science, immunology, and epidemiology, tutored by the late Freeman Cope, MD. Along with Christeene, he has dedicated much of his life to the investigation and evaluation of alternative cancer therapies.

∽

Later that week, I hired Felipe for a full day to make a trip down the coast to Rosarito, a beach resort that is popular with Americans, about thirty minutes from Playas. I had an appointment to meet with Dr. Patrick Vickers, an American chiropractor who has operated the **Northern Baja Healing Center** since 2013, with the assistance of Mexican physicians. Although younger than Gar and Dr. Rogers, Dr. Vickers also has extensive experience with the Gerson Therapy and, upon graduation from chiropractic college, headed to Mexico to work with Charlotte Gerson. The clinic was recently relocated to the top floor of a new oceanfront, high-rise condominium building, just south of the town of Rosarito.

Felipe and I found the building without a problem, but locating the clinic on the twenty-first floor was a bit challenging, as the only signs on the doors warned casual visitors away, stating "Private Property." After a few rings and light knocks at what I hoped to be the right place, the door was opened and I was greeted by Dr. Vickers, whom I recognized from his many video lectures on YouTube and the website chrisbeatcancer.com.

The Northern Baja Healing Center offers what it calls "Advanced Gerson Therapy," and it was truly a beautiful space, with sweeping views of the Pacific from a large balcony that ran the length of the clinic. An immense, sleek kitchen was attended by a very friendly Mexican lady, and the adjacent dining room and lounge/treatment areas had contemporary yet comfortable décor and furnishings, all affording beautiful views. Directly across from the terraces and sitting areas were the ten bedrooms, but I was not able to view any of them, as I was told the patients were in their rooms at that time, doing detoxification therapies. From an adjacent office, a man in a white coat, whom I presumed to be one of the physicians, smiled at me, but I was not introduced to him, and the only other staff I saw was the woman in the kitchen. Dr. Vickers, on the other hand, appeared rushed, and I sensed it would not be opportune to ask him the detailed questions that I had asked other doctors.

From one of the lofty balconies my eyes were drawn to a nearby beach and I asked if it was possible to swim there. Interestingly, Dr. Vickers told me that due to the sodium restriction of the Gerson Therapy, patients are not permitted to swim in salt water. I looked far below to the swimming pool at the edge of the sea and Dr. Vickers said he hoped it would soon be converted to a purification system that did not use chlorine, considered a toxin to be avoided during healing and recovery.

Dr. Vickers told me that his typical patient is someone in their fifties with advanced cancer, and that about 50% have had conventional treatment before coming to the clinic. He has seen an increase in the number of patients who have attempted to treat their own cancer and told me that of those who attempt to do the Gerson Therapy themselves, at home, about 90% fail. He offers a follow-up program after treatment, and companions are encouraged to learn the therapy in order to assist the patient at home. When I asked Dr. Vickers how he responds when patients ask him about his success rate, he said that it was impossible to provide, as success depends on a patient's full compliance with home treatment.

Joy, my acquaintance from the bus tour, had also visited this clinic and met Dr. Vickers. She was impressed with the beautiful, spotlessly clean, and modern treatment environment. Although she did not ultimately select Northern Baja for her cancer treatment, she did feel that it would be a good choice for those who simply wanted to do the Gerson Therapy in an elegant, modern, and comfortable environment. I thought so too, and after leaving the clinic, I wandered the grounds of the condominium complex. I enjoyed the peaceful and natural setting with lush gardens dotted here and there, as well as a walkway that hugged the rocky coastline and led to a small café perched over the sea.

Dr. Vickers has studied the work of Dr. Gerson extensively, and believes, as others do, that prior to his death, Gerson was interested in combining immunotherapies with the Gerson Therapy. In addition to the classic Gerson Therapy and a variety of supplements, Northern Baja states that the clinic provides Coley's toxins, dendritic cell vaccines, immersion hyperthermia, oxygen therapies, intravenous vitamin C, and laetrile in its basic protocol. Chelation and coffee enemas are a component of the detoxification regime. A treatment area contained a Bemer mat, thought to facilitate healing by improving circulation in even the smallest blood vessels, increasing the oxygen content and balancing the electrical charges of the body.

The minimum length of treatment at Northern Baja is two weeks, but at least three weeks is advised for those with cancer. The weekly price in 2017 is just under

$6,000, which includes the complete Gerson Therapy, the additional therapies, and three months of supplements and immunotherapies to take home. Room and board for a companion and transportation to and from the San Diego airport is also included in the base price.

Dr. Vickers has a succinct essay on his website about the powerful forces that restrict health freedom in the U.S. entitled "If it is so good why haven't I heard about it?" It is worth reading, even for those who are not interested in the Gerson Therapy or treatment in Mexico. For more information, visit http://www.gersontreatment.com

◈

Later that day, Felipe drove me just a few miles south to the **Sanoviv Medical Institute**, a large, gleaming white, eight-story building on the ocean. Built on the former site of the mansion that belonged to the Levi Strauss family, American microbiologist Myron Wentz bought the ten-acre property in 2000 with the dream of making it a world-class integrative health center and health resort. I had an appointment for a general tour of the facility and would be having lunch in the dining room with Sanoviv's guests. The guard at the driveway gatehouse checked my name to verify that I was expected and opened the tall solid gates to let Felipe and me through.

I was immediately struck by the elegance of Sanoviv—it was like entering a five-star hotel rather than a hospital. I was assigned to Hector, an engaging, bilingual young man who would serve as my guide for the private tour of the facility. As I walked down wide marbled hallways, I passed sitting areas furnished with antique chairs placed along glass walls that overlooked gardens, the Pacific Ocean, and the resort's swimming pools. I was captivated by the peace and beauty of Sanoviv. Hector told me about its history and about how people come from all over the world for the health retreats and the medical treatments it offers. He said that Sanoviv is particularly popular with people from Europe and Japan, and I did indeed see many Asian guests. All of the guests wore identical beige, organic cotton hospital-like scrubs, a requirement for all of the organic-living treatment programs.

Hector took me to see one of the guestrooms, all of which have terraces overlooking the Pacific. The spacious and spotless room was beautifully decorated and furnished in neutral colors, and featured a separate sleeping area for a companion. The room was complete with a large marbled bath, organic-cotton terry robes, and a small sitting area. The room had a small rebounder, as well as a Chi Machine, both thought to help stimulate lymph flow and increase oxygenation. I saw only this one room, but Hector said that all the rooms contained these same features, although not all offer the separate sleeping area for a companion.

As we wandered down several hallways, I was shown the modern full-service dental suite, chiropractic office, massage rooms, and full-size auditorium, where educational presentations are offered regularly. Hector told me that Sanoviv treats many diseases in addition to cancer and also offers healthy living, detox, and rejuvenation retreats. I was not able to speak with any of the doctors who work within the cancer treatment program, but I was shown the large and spotless ocean view treatment area where the IV therapies are administered. We walked outside to three swimming pools, filled with desalinated, filtered sea water, just behind the path that meanders the length of the property along the sea. My tour concluded at the huge half-circle dining room, with floor-to-ceiling windows that overlook an outdoor dining terrace and the sea beyond.

Lunch was self-service, with a long buffet table that was attended by staff. There was a chicken entrée available, but when I said I was vegetarian, a special mushroom dish was prepared for me. The food was fresh and well presented, but that particular meal was rather bland to my taste, likely by design to suit those with various digestive issues. I left feeling a bit hungry, and later I joked with Felipe that were I a patient at Sanoviv, I would be tempted to sneak out to the taco truck down the road.

Despite my hunger, I thought that it would be a wonderful place to relax and focus on healing for a few weeks. Joy also visited Sanoviv, and as a potential patient, she had the opportunity to meet with one of the physicians. Her confidence in the Sanoviv medical team was not too high, as according to Joy, the doctor told her that they had recently begun using hyperthermia, and presented it as a new, innovative treatment from Europe. Joy was quite aware that hyperthermia has been in use in the clinics in Mexico and Germany for a very long time. Joy did not choose Sanoviv for her treatment, but like me, she was taken with the beauty of it and vowed to return for a rejuvenation retreat someday.

Sanoviv offers many of the same cancer therapies that other clinics offer, such as hyperthermia, intravenous vitamin C and laetrile, dendritic cell vaccines, hyperbaric oxygen, and detoxification therapies. They are one of only two clinics in the area that offer Rigvir, an oncolytic virus therapy. They perform individualized testing and assessment to establish the most appropriate treatment plan, and offer a variety of complementary therapies and spiritual counseling. There is a strong emphasis on nutrition and the diet is mostly plant based, free of gluten, processed foods, and dairy.

I was not able to meet with any of the physicians who treat cancer, and the biographies of the doctors do not include any who appear to have a special focus on or experience with cancer. I spoke with a representative of Sanoviv who told me that each patient is assigned one primary doctor, but that all their doctors are integrative medicine experts and collaborate daily on each patient in the medical programs. She stressed that the treatment of cancer at Sanoviv is constantly evolving, integrating new therapies that have proven to be effective. I can see that the Sanoviv program would be an excellent choice for those who would only be comfortable in very modern and elegant surroundings and feel that their chances of healing would be greater in such a peaceful and protected environment. Sanoviv would also be a great choice for those who have already received conventional cancer treatment that has been declared successful, but who wish to reduce their chances of recurrence, rebuild their immune system, and improve their overall health in beautiful and luxurious oceanfront surroundings.

The cost of the basic cancer treatment program is $29,500 in 2017, which, in addition to room and board, includes three weeks of treatment comprising a variety of consultations, assessments, and classes, many different therapies, and medical spa services. Other therapies, such as Rigvir, dendritic cell vaccines, low-dose chemotherapy, and intravenous turmeric, are offered at additional charges. Companions who stay in the same room with the patient are charged $100 per day for room and board, access to a variety of classes, and use of the Sanoviv facilities. Credit cards are accepted. For more information, visit http://www.sanoviv.com.

CHAPTER 10

A Few More Visits and Other Clinics
Rubio Cancer Center, Hope4Cancer,
and Immunity Therapy Center
CMN-ACT, San Luis de Colorado

One of the first clinics that we visited on the Cancer Control Society tour was the **Rubio Cancer Center**. The Rubio Cancer Center is operated by Dr. Geronimo Rubio, with the assistance of Carolyn Gross, an American who acts as a patient representative and advocate. Several other physicians work at the center, including Dr. Rubio's son. Dr. Rubio is a highly experienced physician who has been treating cancer in an integrative and alternative manner for decades. In the late 1980s, Dr. Rubio established the American Metabolics Institute with an American, William Fry. This clinic was closed in 2004 due to complicated legal issues and, later, Dr. Rubio established his own cancer center after these issues were resolved. The Rubio Cancer Center is now a well-known and respected inpatient treatment facility at the outer edge of Tijuana's commercial district of "Zona Rio," where many of the other clinics are located.

Although the street and surrounding area where the Rubio Cancer Center is located appears rather industrial and unattractive, the building that houses the center appeared very modern and well kept, with a large and prominent "Rubio Cancer Center" sign on the building. The interior was spotlessly clean, with simple but modern furnishings. It is a small facility that treats only nine patients at a time, but Carolyn Gross managed the large size of our group with aplomb. We were first ushered into the surprisingly large dining area, where light refreshments were provided as Carolyn gave us an overview of the treatment philosophy of the clinic. We were guided down a narrow but elegant tiled hallway to view the various treatment rooms on the way to a nicely landscaped garden courtyard with a swimming pool. In order to respect the privacy of several patients who were connected to intravenous drips while lounging around the pool, we did not linger there for long.

Our group was escorted upstairs to a small auditorium/meeting room. There, Dr. Rubio and Dr. Rubio, Jr., welcomed us and gave a fascinating lecture about the various immunotherapies that are a result of their research. Dr. Rubio was clearly passionate about his work and the positive results he has obtained, and answered the many questions that were asked by the group. We were told that they have their own research lab onsite, and it is one of the few in Mexico that is accredited by the government. Only four people from the group were allowed to see the lab due to the risk of contamination by a large group, and I was not one of the four chosen.

The specialty of the Rubio Cancer Center is immunotherapy, but other therapies, supplements, and medications are prescribed, based on an individualized assessment. Low-dose chemotherapy and radiation are used, as indicated. Cancer nutrition and nutrition education are emphasized, and unique to this center is a nutrition plan based on blood type. Treatment is typically three to four weeks, and up to two companions per patient may be accommodated in the patient's room.

Dr. Geronimo Rubio and Carolyn Gross co-authored a book that was published in 2013 entitled "Breaking the Cancer Code: A Revolutionary Approach to Reversing Cancer," which gives a comprehensive overview of the center's philosophies and methods. I was not able to obtain cost information for this clinic. For more information, visit http://www.rubiocancercenter.com.

Another stop on the bus tour was to the **Hope4Cancer Institute**, a clinic that is heavily promoted online and has received a lot of publicity lately. Hope4Cancer has been featured prominently in *The Truth About Cancer* docuseries and is a "verified clinic" listed on the Cancer Tutor website. My attempts to arrange a private visit to Hope4Cancer on a prior trip to Tijuana were not successful. I did not receive responses to the phone messages that I left, and a personal letter of introduction that I sent to the medical director went unanswered. People I met who are "in the know" told me that as a result of all the attention the clinic has received from *The Truth About Cancer* docuseries, the staff had been overwhelmed with the volume of inquiries received.

Hope4Cancer serves both inpatients and outpatients at the clinic in Playas, and outpatients only at a clinic in Cancun, Mexico. The founder and medical director, Dr. Antonio Jimenez, grew up in the United States, and completed his undergraduate education in Texas before attending medical school in Mexico. He states that he has over twenty-five years of experience treating cancer, but it is not clear where he obtained his experience prior to opening the Hope4Cancer Institute. Dr. Jimenez is a frequent speaker at health conferences in the United States, and many of his presentations can be found online, including on YouTube.

I met some people at the Dali Suites who had recently completed a course of treatment at Hope4Cancer and were staying at the hotel overnight before returning home. There were also many people at the hotel who were receiving outpatient treatment at this clinic. I was told that the clinic is perpetually full and often has a waiting list. All the patients I met said that they had learned of Hope4Cancer through the docuseries *The Truth About Cancer* and did not previously know anyone who had been treated there. They all seemed satisfied with their care and treatment, and had confidence in the medical staff.

One gentleman whom I became acquainted with was Greg, a tall, fit, outgoing man in his early seventies, from southern California. Greg had just completed a multiple-week course of inpatient treatment at Hope4Cancer for prostate cancer. Greg was quite satisfied with his treatment and the care that he received, but was concerned that he may have waited too long to seek alternative therapies while he was treated with radiation therapy in California. (I spoke with Greg by phone about a year later, and he was doing very well and had returned to work with reduced hours. He continued to have regular follow-up visits, therapies, and communications with his Hope4Cancer doctors, and was also being monitored by a local physician who was accepting of Greg's choice of treatment and willing to order the tests requested by his Mexican doctors. Greg said he recommended Hope4Cancer, and believed that the patients he knew from the clinic who had not done well or had passed away had waited too long before seeking treatment there.)

On the Cancer Control Society bus tour, Hope4Cancer was our last stop of a long day that began in San Diego for some of us and Los Angeles for most of the participants. Our large group was led down a whitewashed hall into a large, plain meeting room that had rows of chairs set up for us to attend formal presentations by several of the Hope4Cancer doctors who were already seated at a conference table at the front of the room. The back of the large room opened onto an open-air patio, where staff stood by several long buffet tables of food and drink provided for our dinnertime visit.

The presentations by the doctors covered the basics of cancer and alternative cancer treatment as well as information about the various therapies offered at Hope4Cancer. Particularly interesting to me was the presentation by one doctor about the use of a therapy called Recall Healing. Recall Healing, developed by Dr. Gilbert Renaud, of France, and taught mostly in Europe, is a therapy designed to gain access to deep-rooted unconscious emotional traumas that may be interfering with the ability to get well, or could even have triggered cancer or some other disease process. Although most of the doctors I met at the Tijuana clinics acknowledged the role of the psyche and emotions in healing from cancer, especially hope and the strong desire to get well, I was impressed that Hope4Cancer had a structured program in place to address the underlying issues that may fuel the disease. Joy, as well as a few other people on the tour, were impressed with the information presented, and many questions were asked of the doctors. Joy liked this clinic and their philosophy, although the simple, bare-bones nature of the physical environment were not to her liking.

The buffet that was prepared for us was truly amazing. There was a vast array of salads and creative hot vegan dishes, and even fruit- and nut-based low-sugar desserts. I was joined in my praise of the wide array of delicious food by many of the other tour participants. Curiously, when I told a Hope4Cancer patient at the

Dali Suites about the fantastic food, he wryly commented that it didn't sound like what the patients were served. He said that the food was good, but they did not have the great variety of choices I described.

The visit to Hope4Cancer did not include a tour of any of the patient rooms, common areas, or treatment facilities, and I was disappointed that Dr. Jimenez was not present. One of my acquaintances at the Dali Suites said that the clinic was "rough around the edges" throughout, and that the management was working on sprucing up the physical environment. The outside of the clinic building was quite nondescript and anonymous, situated next to local markets and businesses. The clinic sits just across the street from the beach and lively boardwalk of Playas, an ideal location for those who want to exercise outdoors and enjoy the seaside ambiance.

The Hope4Cancer Institute offers a large variety of therapies and treatments, including Rigvir, an oncolytic viral immunotherapy approved by the governments of some European countries. The treatment protocol is formalized in what the Institute labels as the seven key principles of cancer therapy: nontoxic cancer-fighting agents, enhance/optimize immune system, full spectrum nutrition, detoxification, eliminate pathogens, oxygenation, and spiritual and emotional integrity.

Cost information is not published, and treatment costs vary based on each person's individual needs. According to what a few patients who received treatment at Hope4Cancer told me, it is about $40,000 for a three-week course of treatment. Credit cards are not accepted. For more information, visit http://www.hope4cancer.com.

It was just past sunset when our tour ended, and since I was planning to stay in Tijuana for a while, I got my luggage off the bus and prepared to walk the ten minutes over cracked sidewalks to the Dali Suites. I had walked this route many times before during my previous visit, but never alone in the evening, dragging luggage behind me. Along this route was a very old man whom I used to greet daily as he sat in the driveway of his family's home, although he seemed to only begrudgingly respond to me with "Hola" as I passed by. On this evening though, my heart was warmed as his face lit up with a big smile as I passed, and he said, "Hola," and it was clear that he remembered me from my visit a couple of months prior. Other than this pleasant interaction, my experience of walking the streets in Tijuana and Playas were the same as always—no one paid any attention to me.

❦

Since the bus tour only included four clinics, I scheduled a private visit to the **Immunity Therapy Center** in Zona Rio, and had hoped to meet the clinic's founder, Dr. Carlos Bautista. When reviewing this clinic's website, it appeared to offer a variety of therapies and had the relatively reasonable cost of less than $20,000 for a three-week course of treatment. There is little information provided about Dr. Bautista's background and experience, only that he has twenty years of experience treating cancer and had worked in a hospital that offered alternative medicine before opening the Immunity Therapy Center in 2007.

In addition to their informative website, the Immunity Therapy Center is promoted online by Peggy Sue Roberts, a former patient of the clinic who experienced a successful outcome for Stage IV lymphoma after treatment there. On her website, she raves about the wonderful clinic in Mexico, but will not give the name of the clinic until contact information is submitted. I submitted my information, as I was curious about which clinic she was promoting. Shortly thereafter, I received a call from a man who said he was Peggy Sue's nephew. Although I told him the reason for my interest, and that I was not personally seeking treatment, he proceeded with the call in a scripted manner, as if he were trying to sell me on treatment at this clinic.

Just a note: There are some clinics that do give referral fees to third parties to steer business to them, and one clinic director, prior to meeting me, did suggest such a relationship. After meeting me, he must have realized that I was not in the position to refer people to his clinic, nor would I ever recommend a particular clinic for profit, and a business arrangement was not mentioned.

There is also a website, mexicancancerclinics.com, that describes its services as a free patient advocacy and information center that helps people choose the best clinic in Tijuana for their needs. The website, run by Marla Manhart, states that consultations are arranged with the clinic doctor in addition to providing information about therapies, transportation, costs, and filing insurance claims. They may provide a useful service, but they only represent five clinics who likely provide the financial support for the operation of the website.

It was easy to find the Immunity Therapy Center, located in an office building in the center of the bustling Zona Rio district, near upscale hotels, restaurants, and a large shopping mall. I had made a last-minute appointment to visit with Carlos, the clinic's patient representative, but was told that Dr. Bautista was out of town and that another doctor was covering his patients. The reception area was modern and attractively decorated, another medical office that looked like many in the United States. I was ushered to Carlos's office, where he gave me a brochure about the clinic and answered those questions he could, careful not to answer those that were medical in nature. I only had brief glimpses of other areas of the clinic, but it appeared very modern, clean, and well appointed.

According to the materials I was given and the clinic website, Immunity Therapy Center offers a large variety of therapies, including some that are not frequently offered, such as Rife therapy, sonodynamic therapy, and others. The clinic also offers common therapies used in integrative clinics, such as hyperthermia, various intravenous and oxygen therapies, a variety of immunotherapies, low-dose chemo with IPT, and vitamin, enzyme, herbal, and mineral supplements. The published cost of $18,995 for three weeks of treatment, six days per week, includes all therapies, diagnostics, and two meals per day. The clinic states that they accept credit cards. For more information visit http://www.immunitytherapycenter.com.

∽

A hospital that is not located in Tijuana, yet is very close to the United States, is the alternative cancer treatment program at the **Centro Medico del Norte Hospital (CMN)** in San Luis de Colorado, near Yuma, Arizona. CMN is a full-service hospital with an emergency room, intensive care unit, and surgical suites. Within the hospital is an eleven-room inpatient cancer treatment program that offers a large variety of therapies. CMN-ACT (Alternative Cancer Treatment), as the cancer treatment program is called, has received positive attention due to the publicized story of Shannon Knight, who received successful treatment at CMN for Stage IV breast cancer after conventional treatments failed. Although I was not able to visit CMN, I met with the medical director, Edgar Payan, MD, via Skype, spoke with Anna, a CMN-ACT patient representative, and have had several conversations with Shannon Knight.

I found Dr. Payan to be a very warm and gracious man, whose dedication to his patient's wellbeing was very apparent. Dr. Payan has many years of experience treating cancer and is well educated, having received continuing education in the United States, Mexico, and abroad. Although Dr. Payan presented himself with the professionalism of a medical doctor, I also had the sense that I was speaking with a true healer. Dr. Payan recognizes and emphasizes the role of the mind and emotions in recovery, and patients at CMN work with a psychologist to help identify underlying issues that may be barriers to recovery. Therapies, such as Rife therapy, that target the electromagnetic disturbances associated with cancer is one of the offered modalities.

Dr. Payan told me that he does not use the RCGG test, as he doesn't have confidence that testing one natural substance in isolation against the cancer has any value, because many of the natural therapies work in a complementary manner with each other. He feels that even if one particular natural substance scores low on the RCGG test, there is no way to measure how that substance may potentiate other substances to enhance the cytotoxic effect on cancer cells. He echoes the message of many of the physicians that I spoke with in Mexico that it is a multifaceted therapeutic approach that proves most successful.

Unlike many of the other physicians I spoke with, Dr. Payan will not tell potential patients that he can put any specific percentage of patients into remission. He tells them he will do his absolute best, and that he has helped many patients achieve long-term remission, but there are too many individual variables that he has no control over.

Dr. Payan says that about 40% of the patients who come to CMN have Stage IV cancer, and he has seen an increase in the number of patients who seek alternative therapy before submitting to conventional treatment. He says he has also seen an increase in the number of patients coming to CMN from other countries, particularly Australia, the U.K., and a number of European countries.

Although CMN offers a large variety of therapies, treatments such as low-dose chemotherapy and other conventional cancer treatments are not offered; all treatments are non-toxic. Dr. Payan offers most patients autologous stem cell therapy, which he feels is very helpful to support immune function and enhance overall response to the other therapies. Autologous refers to the fact that the patient is the donor of the stem cells, and they are typically removed from the bone marrow of the hip in a short, relatively painless procedure.

Dendritic cell immunotherapy is provided at CMN, but patients are not discharged with the vaccine to administer at home. Dr. Payan says that some patients do experience side effects from the vaccine, and he believes it is safer to administer only while the patient is monitored and under his care.

Dr. Payan is enthusiastic about the recent legalization of medical marijuana in Mexico. He is hopeful that the legal processes to make it available will be in place in about a year, and he plans to offer it. He believes that it will be a valuable adjunct to the therapeutic program, with the benefits of pain management, appetite stimulation, and cytotoxic effects on cancer cells.

The diet for cancer patients at CMN is a balanced plant-based diet, gluten- and dairy-free, with no added sugar or processed foods. Most of the food is organic and a dietician is on staff to modify the diet for individual needs. Dr. Payan is not enthusiastic about the ketogenic diet. Although he acknowledges that cancer consumes a lot of glucose, normal cells consume it as well. He prefers to keep glucose in the diet low, but not as restricted as found in ketogenic diets.

Anna, the patient representative supervisor, presented a picture of CMN as a very nurturing and caring cancer treatment program. She told me that although companions may share a room with the patient for emotional support at no extra cost, it is not always advised. She spoke about how many people with cancer are often focused on the emotional wellbeing of their companion, when it is most beneficial for the patient's healing and recovery to focus on their own wellbeing. Anna said that the hospital is well staffed, and there is no need for companions to help care for the patient, regardless of how ill they might be.

Shannon Knight received treatment at CMN six years ago and has been vocal about the high quality of care and therapy provided there. CMN does not solicit or post any patient testimonials, and Shannon has not received any incentives to share her positive experiences via Facebook or various interviews. Shannon deeply believes that just because CMN was the right choice for her does not automatically mean it might be the right choice for others. Shannon's twin sister, Jessie, also received treatment at CMN for the same type of breast cancer as Shannon had. Jessie is healthy and cancer-free two years later, and shares her sister's satisfaction with the care and treatment she received. Shannon portrayed her stay at CMN as very comforting and nurturing. She told me that every evening, a woman came to her room offering aromatherapy to help with relaxation and sleep, and that staff were always available to provide emotional support.

CMN-ACT is located just fourteen blocks from the Arizona border, in the town of San Luis Rio de Colorado, described as a peaceful town of less than 200,000 people. CMN staff provide complimentary transportation for patients to and from Yuma, Arizona, a thirty-minute drive. CMN offers all the standard alternative and nutritional therapies found in the clinics of Tijuana, such as intravenous vitamin C, laetrile, hyperthermia, hyperbaric oxygen, and many others.

The cost for four weeks of inpatient treatment in 2017 is $39,000, which includes all therapies except any necessary blood transfusions, surgeries, or albumin. This cost also includes stem cell therapy, which is typically an extra charge in the other clinics and hospitals that offer it. Dr. Payan offers email support and monthly Skype calls with patients after discharge. This benefit has no time limit, and is available indefinitely. The cost includes meals and transportation for a companion who shares *the patient's room. Credit cards are not currently accepted, but will be accepted in the very near future. For more information about the CMN-ACT program, visit http://www.CMNact.com.*

Other Clinics

There are other reputable clinics and hospitals with extensive experience treating cancer that I was unable to visit, or speak with their physicians, and which I hope to include in future travels. Their exclusion from this book does not imply that they are not excellent treatment choices worthy of consideration.

⚬

Dr. Isai Castillo of the **CIPAG Clinic** is quite well known, and is particularly popular with people from Canada. I have heard that treatment costs are reasonable and that many Amish patients receive treatment at this clinic. Dr. Castillo established CIPAG in 1984 after working at numerous other hospitals, including the original Hospital del Mar with Ernesto Contreras, the Gerson Clinic, and the Bio-Medical/Hoxsey Clinic. CIPAG is an outpatient clinic in Tijuana's Zona Rio that offers a large variety of therapies and has its own pharmacy, laboratory, and X-ray facilities. My friend Grace, from the Dali Suites, had a consultation with Dr. Castillo about adding on a therapy that was not offered at St. Andrews Clinic, and she told me, "I got a very good feeling from Dr. Castillo's place, and the patients raved about him. They were Christians to the core and very caring." For more information, visit http://www.drcastillo.com.

⚬

The **Europa Institute of Integrated Medicine**, located only a few blocks from the border, in Tijuana's Zona Rio, was established in 1989 by Dr. Sonia Rodriguez and her American late husband, Dr. Jeffrey Freeman. On the clinic's website, the cancer treatment goals are described as an ongoing process to remove toxins, replenish nutrients, restore circulation and detoxification capability, balance biochemistry, strengthen the immune system, reduce free

179

radicals, and address the underlying subconscious issues that drive everything. The Europa Institute states that it is a Christian clinic and strives to keep costs reasonable. The clinic offers a variety of therapies for cancer and other chronic illnesses. For more information, visit http://www.europainstitute.org.

∽

Mentioned previously, **Issels Immuno-Oncology** has an inpatient cancer treatment program in the Angeles Hospital in the Zona Rio district of Tijuana, as well as an outpatient clinic in Santa Barbara, California. From my conversations with patients who had inquired about treatment at Issels, the cost is quite high—possibly the highest cost of all the treatment choices in Tijuana. For more information, visit http://www.issels.com.

∽

Angeles Hospital in Tijuana's Zona Rio is a large, modern hospital that is reported to maintain the high standards of many of the best hospitals worldwide. Within Angeles Hospital is an inpatient integrative cancer treatment program that offers a full range of alternative and integrative treatments. On staff is Dr. Donato Perez Garcia, known for his expertise in low-dose chemotherapy with IPT (insulin potentiation therapy), and whose grandfather first developed this therapy. For more information, visit http://www.cancertreatment.mx.com or http://www.donatoperezgarcia.com.

CHAPTER 11
Success Rates, Doctors, Costs, and More

When considering A/I treatment in Mexico or in any country, including the United States, there are obvious questions and concerns that someone would have as they consider straying from the norm of conventional treatment. Likely, the biggest concern is: *Will it work?* The second is likely: *How much does it cost, and can I afford it?* Other important questions include those about insurance reimbursement, the qualifications of the doctors, the type and amount of follow-up care that will be necessary, and how to choose a clinic or doctor. In this section I will address these questions and concerns, with the understanding that there are no absolute answers to these inquiries.

Success Rates

Often people refer to the survival data provided by the SEER statistics that show five-year survival rates based on site and stage of cancer at diagnosis. SEER (Surveillance Epidemiology and End Results) is a program of the National Cancer Institute that collects data on cancer cases from various locations and sources throughout the United States, and provides a report of the most recent cancer incidence, mortality, survival, prevalence, and lifetime risk statistics. According to the National Cancer Institute, SEER coverage includes only approximately 28% of the U.S. population, including 26% of African Americans, 38% of Hispanic Americans and 50% of Asian Americans, among other provided race and ethnicity breakdowns.[1]

Survival rates, regardless of who is providing them, are simply statistical averages, and do not account for the varying types of cancers within a specific diagnosis, for example, in breast cancer where treatment and survival are influenced by hormone receptor status and the particular histology (microscopic structure) of the cancer. Survival rates also do not reflect the characteristics of the person with the cancer, such as age and overall health status, or lifestyle issues such as smoking, diet, stress, sleep, and exercise levels.

Certainly, many of those who embark upon an intensive recovery plan after treatment, conventional or otherwise, are likely to have a higher rate of five-year survival and long-term remission than any official statistic would show. Research is just starting to provide evidence that lifestyle changes do make a difference in avoiding cancer recurrence after treatment, but to my knowledge there is no research comparing the treatment outcomes of those who embark upon lifestyle changes with those who don't, while they are in treatment.

Shannon Knight, the stage IV breast cancer survivor mentioned in the previous chapter who received successful treatment from CMN hospital, in Mexico, wrote a blog post titled "Cancer Treatment Success Rate: The Truth." (The full post can be found at http://www.shannonknight.com). Shannon writes:

> One of the most common questions to a cancer treatment facility from a cancer patient is, "What is the success rate?" Can you imagine what would happen if a doctor turned that question around on patients and asked, "What do you think your success rate is? What is your plan in this healing partnership?" Patients do have choices of how they treat their body; the doctors are not solely responsible for a patient's health.
>
> Take into consideration the types of drugs a patient has taken, how many rounds of chemotherapy or radiation they have received, surgery, pain management, diet, alcohol, cigarettes, environment, or overall health. A patient's chance of success is also going to be determined by what she does at home for self-treatment. He [the doctor] is relying on you as much as you are relying on him. The doctor cannot do many of these things "for you" that make a big difference in your success. You have more power over success than you realize. Cancer treatment is a

partnership and doctors cannot make promises. Educating ourselves on the treatments recommended is imperative. We need to do a lot of research on a drug or therapy before taking it. We must look at the pros and cons. If we are choosing an alternative approach, is it the very best and is it aggressive enough?"

The role of compliance and individual variability when considering the success of alternative cancer treatment is addressed by the late Dr. Nicholas Gonzalez and Dr. Linda Isaacs in an article entitled "Statistics: Why Meaningful Statistics Cannot Be Generated from a Private Practice."[2] Their article also discussed the complexity of determining survival rates, and they voiced their opinion that survival rates compared to SEER data have very minimal value. The authors stated that even the highly funded American cancer centers such as M.D. Anderson and Memorial Sloan Kettering cannot provide success rates on various types of cancers. The authors state: "Not only are there different histological types, each carrying with it a different prognosis, but to complicate the matter, pathologists divide each specific cell type into grades, another measure of aggressiveness based on the appearance of the cancer cells under the microscope. This classification scheme usually breaks down into 3 categories: well differentiated (least aggressive), moderately differentiated (moderately aggressive), and poorly differentiated (most aggressive), each in turn associated with a different prognosis. For each, different treatments might be suggested." Dr. Gonzalez and Isaacs also stated their opinion that prior therapy affects the ultimate prognosis and outcome, and that the damage caused by previous conventional treatments (that can also create a more aggressive form of cancer) is often the cause of death rather than the cancer.

To my knowledge, the only A/I program in Tijuana that compares its survival rates to SEER data is Oasis of Hope. Oasis of Hope has collected their own data for many years, and states that its survival rates for Stage IV cancers are up to three times higher than those achieved with conventional treatment. On an Oasis of Hope webpage you will find charts comparing Oasis of Hope survival rates with 2007 SEER data.

Although Oasis has not updated the statistics on this page, I found that the 2007 and most recent 2016 SEER data are not very different. The five-year SEER survival rate for Stage IV breast cancer was 24% in 2007 and 26.9% in 2016. Oasis of Hope states that its survival rate is 45% for those who have previously had conventional treatment, and 75% for those whose first treatment was at Oasis of Hope. The current SEER data for Stage IV melanoma five-year survival is 20%; Oasis states that its rate is 75%. I can't speak to how accurate its data collection is, but Oasis of Hope has likely treated the largest number of Stage IV patients over the longest period of time of any of the other A/I Tijuana clinics.

Unfortunately, there is no absolute way to know if any given course of treatment, conventional or A/I, will be successful for a particular patient. In conventional oncology, there is a reliance on data provided by clinical trials, usually funded by pharmaceutical companies who stand to profit from a successful outcome. It is well documented that the drug trials funded by pharmaceutical companies are more likely to result in positive outcomes for the drug being tested (see chapter 5).

As most of the people who seek out A/I treatment in Mexico are Stage IV patients who have been given a terminal diagnosis, with only palliative chemotherapy or radiation therapy offered, A/I treatment might be their only hope. Many of the doctors I spoke with in Mexico were emphatic that if A/I treatment is received before conventional treatment for metastatic disease, success rates are higher. It is not just Mexican doctors who make this claim. My studies of the work of American A/I doctors reveal the same opinion. This makes sense to me, considering that chemotherapy and radiation are known to increase the aggressiveness of cancer, and are largely ineffective against cancer stem cells. Chemotherapy and radiation are also known to damage the immune system, so how could treatments that increase the aggressiveness of cancer, while damaging the person's resistance to further metastasis and infections, possibly lead to any kind of positive outcome?

Costs and Health Insurance

The costs of A/I treatment in Mexico can seem very high, even out of reach, to many people, resulting in some sources accusing these clinics and doctors of charging exorbitant fees that take advantage of desperate people. It is helpful to examine the costs of medical care in the United States and compare these costs to what is being charged in the Tijuana A/I clinics to see whether clinics in Mexico are really charging exorbitant fees or it only seems exorbitant because insurance won't cover non-standard treatment. The average hospital stay in the United States costs about $2,000 per day, according to Beckers Hospital review data,[3] and healthcare.gov states that the average cost of a three-day hospital stay is around $30,000.[4]

An exact comparison is difficult to make, but consider that three to four weeks of inpatient treatment at CMN Hospital, International Bio Care, or Integrative Whole Health Clinic costs $1,000–1,400 per day, including most treatments *and* room and board for both patient and a companion. Outpatient care at a clinic such as the San Diego or Stella Maris comes in at about $1,000 per day, including hotel expenses.

The average net costs of cancer care in the United States have increased steadily, and the National Cancer Institute estimates that the cost of care for the last year of life of a person with cancer ranges from about $60,000–140,000, depending on the type of cancer.[5] Estimating that an individual would be responsible for deductibles, co-payments, and uncovered services of about 10–20%, this could represent anywhere from $6,000 to $28,000 in out-of-pocket expenses.

According to The American Society of Clinical Oncology, newly approved cancer drugs cost an average of $10,000 per month, with some therapies costing $30,000 per month.[6] Patients typically pay 20–30% out of pocket for drugs, so a year's worth of new drugs would cost $24,000 to $36,000, in addition to other expenses such as deductibles and co-pays for other treatment costs.

Clearly, cancer treatment is very expensive. What makes treatment in Mexico and in all A/I clinics, including those in the United States, seem more expensive is the fact that health insurance does not cover therapies that are not FDA approved and considered the standard of care for the treatment of cancer. Some insurance plans will not cover any expenses incurred outside of the United States, even if FDA approved, while other insurance companies will.

It is very difficult to navigate the issues associated with obtaining medical care at out-of-network providers. Many recommend AMHA, The American Medical Health Alliance, a Houston company that helps patients receive the maximum reimbursement for costs at an A/I clinic. AMHA provides a free evaluation of a patient's insurance benefits and charges a fee of 20% of any reimbursement they obtain. For more information, visit http://www.amhabilling.com.

Obtaining Funds to Pay for Treatment

It is truly a sad phenomenon that despite having health insurance, such insurance does not allow for personal choice of treatment, especially in the case of most Stage IV cancers where the standard of care is acknowledged to be merely palliative rather than curative, and the cost of this care is so high. Although some people may get some of their costs from an A/I clinic reimbursed by insurance companies, these expenses would only be for those diagnostics, medications, or treatments that are a part of FDA-approved standard treatment.

I had a heartbreaking conversation about financing with a middle-aged woman I met in Tijuana who was receiving treatment for cancer that was considered terminal. She was unmarried, and had arranged her estate so that her modest assets would pass directly to her two adult children, rather than through a will that would go through the probate process and result in an estate that creditors could collect from, upon her death. She shared with me how difficult it was to face these financial decisions when she was also facing her own mortality. She maxed out her available credit to pay for treatment and rationalized that if she achieved remission, she could eventually pay it off, but if she died, a large wealthy bank would instead be stuck with the bill.

Personal loans and home refinancing are obvious possibilities of obtaining the funds for treatment, but, sadly, for those with cancer that is deemed terminal, the financial ripple effects on surviving family must be considered, should treatment not lead to long-term remission. Since several of the clinics do accept credit cards, those who are short on cash but have adequate credit limits to cover treatment could choose this option.

Many patients who want to raise funds for A/I treatment successfully use the crowdfunding approach on sites such as GoFundMe.com. Using these online sites to raise a significant sum of money requires a bit of marketing effort to target a patient's contacts, church, workplace, and other sources, and is often undertaken by a supportive family member or friend.

When all else fails, some patients who meet certain requirements can enter into a viatical settlement, where the sale of a policy owner's existing life insurance policy to a third party for more than its cash value, but less than its death benefit, provides the policy owner a lump sum. These are available to those who are chronically ill and unable to care for themselves, or to those who are terminally ill, with a life expectancy of two years or less. This option for obtaining the money for A/I treatment is obviously an extreme choice for many people, as if treatment is not successful, funds that would have benefited their surviving family have now been sacrificed.

Medical Qualifications

There is a difference in the basic education between physicians in the United States and in Mexico. In the United States, an undergraduate degree is followed by four years of medical school. Medical school graduates must do a one-year internship to qualify for licensure, but most do this internship as a part of a residency in a specialty that requires three to seven additional years of supervised practice. The more advanced specialties, such as oncology, also require an additional year or two of a fellowship that allows them to become board-certified specialists. All told, most doctors in the United States receive eleven or more years of education following graduation from high school.

In contrast, entry into a medical school in Mexico does not require an undergraduate degree. After four years of medical school, to obtain licensure, Mexican physicians must then complete one year of a medical social-service internship in a government-operated clinic or hospital in an underserved area. Many Mexican physicians establish private practices or take jobs in a hospital after the required year of internship.

Many of the doctors in the A/I clinics in Tijuana have, however, completed undergraduate degrees prior to medical school, and some have done post-medical school residencies, as is typical in the American system of physician education. Some have pursued advanced training in other sciences, such as nutrition, or have traveled to Europe to study and train in therapies related to A/I cancer treatment.

All of the medical directors of the more well-known and respected Mexican cancer clinics/hospitals have extensive experience treating cancer, typically gained by working alongside other experienced physicians and attending educational programs outside of Mexico, most often in Europe. Since an A/I approach to treating cancer has been in practice in Tijuana for about fifty years, much of this experience and expertise has been passed down to the younger generation of physicians. Many of the more mature and experienced physicians were treating patients with an A/I approach before the contemporary movement toward A/I treatment in the U.S. had even been born.

Even in the U.S.-based A/I clinics, few doctors are board-certified oncologists, although all have board certification in some specialty, such as internal medicine or family practice. The primary focus of conventional oncology training is in the delivery and management of chemotherapy or radiation therapy, and as this is not a primary focus in A/I treatment, it has little relevance to the ability to provide treatment in a paradigm that uses largely nontoxic therapies.

Although I did not research to confirm the stated backgrounds of the physicians who work in or operate the clinics described in this book, I chose not to include any clinics whose lead physicians do not state qualifications that indicate a high degree of experience and expertise. Many of the larger clinics and hospitals employ multiple doctors, often newer doctors who work under the supervision of more experienced physicians. If you are interested in treatment at any of the clinics, I suggest you ask the physician directly about his or her qualifications and experience, as well as inquire about those of any other physicians who would be involved in your care. I have found the physicians in Tijuana to be very open and willing to discuss their background, treatment philosophy, and the therapies they offer.

The vast majority of doctors in the A/I clinics offer a free consultation, either by phone, Skype, or in person, and this is a recommendation I would make. In addition, research has shown that the doctor-patient relationship itself acts as a powerful placebo,[7] making the choice of a doctor with whom one feels a sense of trust, hope, and confidence an extremely important factor in treatment success.

Choosing

If one is seriously considering treatment in one of the A/I clinics, I highly recommend visiting these clinics and doctors if finances and health allow, as my acquaintance Joy did, and as did others whom I met on the bus tour. Joy also visited clinics in the United States and had Skype calls with doctors in Germany before deciding on where she would go for treatment. Joy was emphatic that having confidence in the treatment and doctor, as well as addressing the underlying emotional issues related to cancer, were crucial to her successful treatment.

Although the physical environments of all the clinics I visited would be acceptable to me, and the run-down nature of some of the areas of Tijuana would not influence my decision, these were factors that weighed heavily in Joy's preferences and eventual choices. She ultimately chose two different American A/I doctors, but also went to the Bio-Medical Center and began the Hoxsey treatment. (Joy notified me in October 2017 that all of her cancer markers were now normal, and one doctor told her she saw no evidence of cancer in her body.)

For the visits to clinics not featured on the bus tour, Joy and her friend located a taxi service that provided an English-speaking driver who picked them up at their San Ysidro, California, hotel and took them across the border for her appointments at the clinics. This was expensive, as taxi services must have special permits that allow them to operate in both the United States and Mexico. Joy said she found it a very relaxing way to visit the clinics, as the bilingual driver knew exactly where they were going and she would not have been comfortable crossing the border independently and hiring a taxi in Mexico.

My friend Grace, whom I met at the Dali Suites and who had treatment at St. Andrews clinic, made her decision after speaking with both Ralph Moss, who offers phone consultations to help patients individualize their cancer treatment, and Gar Hildenbrand of the Gerson Research Organization. She had not visited the clinic prior to arriving for treatment but was familiar with the area from a prior trip to visit a friend who was receiving treatment for other reasons in Tijuana. A New Yorker in her fifties who lives in a modern and comfortable home, Grace was not at all bothered by the sometimes run-down environments of Tijuana and Playas, and despite not speaking Spanish, she made several friends among the locals. Not only did she feel comfortable traveling around the area, on one weekend she made over one hundred sandwiches before Felipe was to take her to an area where people were homeless and hungry. She described the people as being polite and grateful when she and Felipe, with tears in his eyes, distributed the food.

Some people may look to the patient testimonials that are sometimes present on a clinic or hospital's website to get some sense of reassurance that the treatment program will result in success. These are not limited to Mexican alternative clinic websites; they can be found on the websites of alternative clinics and large, well-known cancer centers in the U.S. as well. It is important to remember that these are marketing tools, particularly the professionally produced video testimonials, and although the clinic may offer excellent treatment, no one can ever guarantee that one person will achieve the same results as another. There are ethical concerns about this practice, and it is possible that some people who feel sick and vulnerable may feel pressured to comply with a request to provide these testimonials, especially if financial incentives are involved. Although I don't know if Mexican physicians take any form of the Hippocratic Oath, close to all medical school graduates in the U.S. declare some version of it. The modern version of this oath includes two sentences that relate to this issue: *I will respect the privacy of my patients, for their problems are not disclosed to me that the world may know. Most especially must I tread with care in matters of life and death.*

Shannon Knight is very passionate about this subject, and wrote an essay, which she posted on Facebook, sharing her thoughts about why these testimonials are not helpful for potential patients, and are ethically wrong.

> *Every doctor upon graduation from medical school makes a promise to act in the best interest of their patients and to protect patient privacy. This most treasured promise that is made before beginning their medical practice is "The Hippocratic Oath." This oath brings a feeling of reassurance that throughout our lifetimes, our chosen physicians will always have our health and best interests at heart. I have seen that oath thrown away by many physicians because of the potential of cancer patients bringing in big business for them. No matter which way you look at the marketing strategy of patient video testimonials on cancer hospital websites, it comes out the same way. It's just wrong and represents a broken promise that physicians made when they swore that oath. Even worse is the recent discovery of deceased patient video testimonials which remain on the hospital/clinic's website long after the patient has passed away. Whether it has been due to a gross oversight and neglect to maintain their website, or an intentional use for marketing purposes, it puts the patient's family through a potentially daunting experience. I can't help but wonder what emotional impact this has on the grieving process of the families and other loved ones.*

Independent reviews, provided by patients who have achieved a lasting remission, may have more value than those found on the websites of the hospitals or clinics. These reviews may be useful to obtain information about how a patient felt about their care, details about the physical environment, treatments, and the attention they received from their doctor, but still give no guarantee that another person will have the same results.

Regardless of a clinic or hospital's notoriety or marketing strategies, I believe that having confidence in the medical team and the treatments should be the core of the decision-making process. How easily can a phone/Skype or in-person consultation be set up with a doctor to discuss receiving treatment? Do your calls with the facility or doctor feel like you are being given a hard sell, or is authentic concern expressed? As with any major decision, research about the treatments, doctors, and clinics, combined with a deeper intuitive sense of what is right for each individual, may be the most useful strategy.

Follow-up/Aftercare

Some clinics have follow-up programs included in the cost of treatment that may allow a patient to speak about their concerns to a doctor at any point in the future, while others have expectations that patients will return after a certain period of time for additional therapies and/or follow-up exams. Also important to consider is whether the physician will be willing to speak with health care providers in a patient's hometown, and share records and recommendations for diagnostic tests, bloodwork, or additional therapies with that provider. It is unlikely that an American oncologist would agree to have this sort of communication, but integrative or functional medicine doctors and naturopaths may be willing to collaborate.

Although some people achieve complete remission after only weeks of treatment, like Bailey O'Brien (chapter 1), whose treatment lasted a mere three weeks, for most patients, treatment is a longer process. It is very important to have a doctor close to home to monitor one's progress. Depending on geographic location, it can sometimes be challenging to find a doctor who is open to alternatives for treating cancer. (For help locating integrative doctors in the United States, see Appendix B.)

There are a variety of laboratory tests that extend beyond the standard cancer marker blood tests performed by conventional oncology that can reveal progression or remission of disease. An example is the OncoStat Plus test, done by RCGG labs, and often called the "Greece" test, that can determine the numbers of circulating tumor cells and cancer stem cells. (For more information on the variety of lab tests that can be used to monitor progress, I recommend the book *Cancer Free, Are You Sure?* by Jenny Hrbacek, RN.)

Cancer Treatment Is a Business

Alternative cancer treatment is a business in Tijuana, just as conventional cancer treatment is a business in the United States. The Tijuana clinics have been described by critics as charging exorbitantly high prices and making unrealistic promises about curing cancer. In my experience with the clinics I visited, this was not apparent. None of the doctors I spoke with promised cures, and all of them felt that the majority of terminally ill patients could at least be helped with an improvement in quality of life, with 50% or more achieving a durable (lasting or long-term) remission. Just like any other business, the clinics have operating costs, and many of the therapies are expensive, having to be imported from other countries. In addition, many of the clinics use sophisticated diagnostic and treatment equipment that must be imported from Europe or the United States, and some therapies, such as the various vaccines, are made in specialized labs.

It is important to remember that conventional cancer treatment in the U.S. is also a hugely profitable business that generates billions of dollars each year. The ethics of the cancer industry in the U.S. is often questioned, with two practices being of particular concern.

First, oncologists in private practices make most of their income by buying chemotherapy drugs wholesale and selling them to patients at marked-up prices, a practice called "buy and bill" that is unique to oncology. There is pressure to make money by selling medications that carry a high price tag rather than using an equally effective but less expensive drug.[8] Physician Robert Pearl, writing for *Forbes*, states: "[B]uy and bill creates a conflict between the medical interests of the patient and the economic interests of the physician."[9]

Second, adding to the concern about financial and pharma influence on the prescribing practices of oncologists, a recent study found that oncologists were more likely to prescribe drugs from pharma companies from whom they received payments. The study, presented at the 2017 American Society of Clinical Oncology Annual Meeting, found that physicians who were paid by pharmaceutical companies for meals, talks, and travel had higher odds of prescribing those companies' drugs to treat the two cancer types that were being studied, regardless of the cost and side-effect profile of the drug. For this study, the treatment options were equivalent in effectiveness, but the authors considered that this same influence of pharma payments may hold true for situations when the treatment choices are not equally effective, an even larger ethical concern.[10]

CHAPTER 12
The Perfect World of Cancer Treatment

In a perfect world, it would not be necessary for a person with cancer to drain their finances and leave their home, family, pets, and friends to travel to another city or country to receive the treatment of their choosing. In this perfect scenario, oncologists would be fully aware of the benefits of therapies and lifestyle changes that focus on the restoration of health of the person who has cancer, rather than just be experts on how to try to eradicate tumors using highly profitable pharmaceuticals. Oncologists would be free to openly speak about other ways of treating cancer and/or minimizing the side effects of their treatments, they would be aware of the research that supports other therapies, and they would have a network of integrative colleagues with whom they would collaborate and refer patients, according to a patient's choice. In "the land of the free," that freedom would extend to our choice of health care options, and health insurance policies would reflect our right to choose.

In this ideal health care world, pharmaceutical companies would no longer have the freedom to engage in aggressive tactics to influence government health care policy, research outcomes, and the clinical practice of physicians. No longer could they forcefully market their most profitable drugs directly to consumers. To boot, a portion of their astronomical profits would have to be used to study nontoxic therapies that have been proven safe and effective in the clinical experience of qualified health professionals, with the oversight of researchers who have no financial interest in the results. Oncologists would then have the data they need to adhere to the principles of "evidence-based medicine," and make referrals to naturopaths, nutritionists, and integrative doctors.

I could go on in my utopian musings about a perfect health care system, but we all know that this ideal is unlikely in our lifetimes. In the meantime, those of us who do not want to subject ourselves to the harsh treatments of mainstream medicine, for whatever reasons, must do our own research and patch together our own individualized treatment and recovery plan. There are many resources to help someone with cancer sift through all the possibilities, including a growing number of cancer coaches and consultants like myself who are health professionals, or who are people who have personally been through cancer and cancer treatment.

Those who have the financial means and live in an area where A/I treatment is available with an experienced and qualified medical professional have a far easier choice than those who must travel and assume greater financial risk to take advantage of a potential to save their lives. I can imagine that most people would prefer to stay in their home country rather than go to Mexico, or even Europe, a more expensive option. Fortunately, there are now many A/I clinics in the U.S. using many standard A/I therapies, as well as innovative approaches that legal regulations allow. However, there are significantly greater legal limitations on the practice of American A/I doctors, and therapies such as intravenous mistletoe, laetrile, Coley's fluids, and others cannot be administered. Appendix B lists some of the better-known clinics and doctors in the U.S., but at present, I know only of two patients' experiences at one of these clinics. My knowledge of the cost differences between the American A/I clinics and the clinics I visited in Tijuana has been obtained only through conversations I had with patients in Mexico, and it is my understanding that treatment at the American clinics is far more expensive. I welcome feedback about patient experiences at these clinics so that I may help others with this information.

For those who may wonder, I don't have an easy answer to the question "Would you go to Mexico for cancer treatment?" I have already said that, post-diagnosis, I would likely take a trip to the Bio-Medical Center to begin the Hoxsey treatment while I considered other strategies to add to a recovery plan. The relatively low investment of money and time, combined with the glowing unsolicited patient testimonials over the past fifty years, would be enough for me to hop on a plane. For the many people who have been consuming the standard American diet, I consider making an immediate dietary change the most important first step while considering treatment options.

I view the three or four weeks of treatment at most of the Tijuana clinics as just one piece of an overall treatment and recovery plan, and believe that this treatment could be very helpful to jumpstart the journey to remission for many people. Although some people are in a position to stay in Mexico for longer periods of time, or make frequent treatment visits, it is not possible for others. It is unrealistic to expect that a few weeks of treatment will result in a long-term remission if the person is not willing to do the necessary work on their own, when they return home. This may involve following their aftercare plan to the letter, monitoring their progress with an integrative health care practitioner and/or open-minded oncologist, and making permanent lifestyle changes—body, mind, and spirit.

For those who have less advanced cancer and received conventional treatment that has been deemed successful, a few weeks at a clinic could be very helpful to restore health and immune function and minimize the chance of recurrence as well as the secondary cancers sometimes caused by chemotherapy and radiation. It is known that by the time even a low-grade, localized tumor is diagnosed, there are cancer cells circulating in the bloodstream. It is an unfortunate fallacy of tumor-focused medicine to think that surgery "got it all," and we know that the chemo or radiation often advised following surgery is unlikely to eliminate rogue cancer stem cells, and often makes the cancer more aggressive and resistant to further treatment with chemo.

For those with advanced Stage III and Stage IV cancers who have been told that their condition is terminal, please believe that it is possible to survive and thrive long term, so don't give up hope. With the exception of a very few types of cancer, conventional treatments are not helpful for metastasized cancer, and many people suffer—and some die—from the treatments rather than the cancer. There are so many people with advanced cancers who have defied their doctor's prognosis, and their stories are inspirational and often miraculous. There are even many people who have achieved remission without spending tens of thousands of dollars at A/I clinics, but most have worked with local practitioners, made major shifts in all areas of their life, and have been very disciplined about following their recovery plan. It is my sincere wish that anyone with cancer who reads this book will soon hear what many others have heard from their oncologist: "I can't explain how your cancer has disappeared, but keep doing what you're doing."

EPILOGUE
Vivi's Story

"In a way, we have more faith in the power of cancer to kill us than we have faith in the power of miracles, the power of infinite possibilities." Marianne Williamson, from the film Heal

My friend Vivi, who was sent home to "get her affairs in order" after the recurrence of metastatic malignant melanoma, had always been a bit of a rebel. Instead of passively accepting the death sentence the doctors had given her, she envisioned a different reality. She decided that the place to begin was with her negative thoughts. Vivi told me that for years her mind had been filled with thoughts of anger toward the injustices and insults of her life experiences, and her stressful job and the initial cancer diagnosis only added another layer of anger.

Vivi began school not long after desegregation, and as an African-American woman, she had traumatic memories of cruel discrimination as a child that were later easily brought back to the surface in her adult life. Her mother had died when she was quite young, and despite feeling lucky that her father later married a woman who cared for Vivi as if she were her own child, the grief over the loss of a parent stayed with her. She married young and eventually divorced, describing her husband as physically and emotionally abusive. Vivi once told me that she had a "whole lot of forgiving to do," and set a course for herself to begin the process.

Although psychologist Kelly A. Turner published her book *Radical Remission* long after Vivi set out on her healing quest, I can see that Vivi implemented many of the strategies that Turner discovered in her research of people who defied a terminal diagnosis. Vivi's first strategy was to take control of her own health, not relying on any outside authority to dictate what path she should take. Vivi began to deepen her spirituality, and became involved with a Buddhist temple as well as a church that focused on changing negative beliefs. She found the yoga classes, Reiki, and massage healing sessions offered at Cornucopia House very helpful in reducing stress and increasing mindfulness of her negative thoughts. She began reading all sorts of books about healing, changing negative thoughts, and forgiveness, and began a meditation practice. Vivi found that her intuition increased through these practices, and she was better able to make decisions and move forward with her healing plan. Vivi changed her diet somewhat, basically just eliminating much of the meat and junk food she had been eating. She tried to include more fruits and vegetables, but did not adopt any rigid dietary rules.

Due to the severe lymphedema (swelling) of her leg and her grave prognosis, Vivi was eligible for disability payments, although they barely covered her basic expenses. Her stress was reduced by not having to work in a highly stressful hospital job, but finances became a big concern. Money was very tight, and Vivi was not able to afford some of the therapies that she believed would be important to her healing and recovery.

In a twist of fate that was both a blessing and a curse, money showed up from an unlikely source. After Vivi's second surgery, she felt much worse than she had after her first surgery. She experienced much more pain in her abdomen, as well as her leg. She had the nurse call the doctor during the night to see her, as she was convinced something was wrong. Her concerns were dismissed, but her pain medication was increased. In the morning when a group of doctors came to see her, she again expressed her concern that something wasn't right, and relayed the symptoms she had that she had not experienced after her first surgery. Again, these concerns were dismissed with explanations that the cancer had been more advanced and that the surgery was longer this time. I don't remember how many months had elapsed before she went back to her oncologist for a check-up and a routine scan of some sort. The scan revealed that her left ureter still had a clamp in place which should have been removed at the conclusion of the surgery. Her oncologist told her that her left kidney was now a non-functional shell. Vivi told me that one of the chemotherapy drugs that had been offered to her after the surgery was one that carried a high risk of kidney toxicity, and Vivi was very glad that she had declined.

In an effort to avoid a lawsuit, her case was handled by an arbitrator, who was to negotiate a settlement between Vivi and the hospital. A month or so later, a settlement was reached and Vivi received a large sum of money. Now, with some money in the bank, Vivi was able to do those things she felt would be helpful. She began receiving care from a local acupuncturist and herbalist who had experience helping people with cancer. She could now receive more frequent lymphedema treatments than were covered by her insurance, which greatly increased her comfort and enabled her to take long meditative walks in a nearby park. Vivi attended classes to become certified in Reiki and Healing Touch, two energy healing practices. She invested in art supplies, and reignited her passion for painting that had been buried for years, rediscovering the joy of creativity.

Vivi told me that the anger and other negative emotions that she had tried to suppress for years were a type of cancer, eating away at her enjoyment of life and growing out of control. She began doing a classic form of loving kindness meditation, sending thoughts of well-being and peace to herself and to those who had angered her. Little by little, she began to forgive. Although Vivi had always been a social person, she cut ties with those she found to be negative and instead spent time with people who nurtured her spirituality. The people she chose to spend time with helped her increase her intuition, explore her reasons for living, and supported her in releasing old emotional baggage. She began volunteering at Cornucopia House, providing energy healing to others with cancer, which she found deepened her spiritual connection and strengthened her life force even further.

It was clear that Vivi was giving her whole being a message of life and joyful thriving. Her whole personality and outlook shifted in a very perceptible manner. She laughed even louder, smiled even more, and the hard, angry edges softened into compassion for others. She had a general love of life, and her spiritual practice took center stage in her life.

According to the American Cancer Society, if diagnosed today, patients with metastatic malignant melanoma have a 10–15% chance of surviving ten years, but when found on the sole of the foot, as it was in Vivi's case, the survival time is shorter. In addition, melanoma is uncommon among African-Americans, but when it does occur, survival times tend to be shorter still.

Vivi lived a fulfilling and healthy life for just over ten years before her life was interrupted by many stressful events. As she had been cancer-free for ten years, she lost her disability payments and had to return to work. She chose a less stressful job than she previously had, but for a sixty-year-old woman who still had some pain and weakness in her leg, it was challenging. Shortly thereafter, her stepmother, with whom Vivi had remained very close, passed away. There were many disagreements within the family about her stepmother's possessions, and Vivi's angry thoughts took over. Vivi simmered with rage as she attempted to cope with all of these stressors.

Vivi developed a painful cough and felt so ill that she asked me to drive her to a doctor's appointment. Despite her history, the doctor dismissed it as a virus and did not order any diagnostic tests. A few weeks later, when the cough didn't subside, a chest X-ray was done, revealing the worst possible news—there was cancer in her lung. Later, in the hospital, bone metastases were found. Vivi went home from the hospital but quickly declined, and she passed away within a few weeks.

Writing this story of Vivi more than ten years after her death still saddens me, and I wish it had a happier ending. But Vivi's life was joyfully prolonged far beyond the prognosis given by her doctors. She had ten more years to be a part of her grandchildren's lives, and she enriched the lives of her family, friends, and those she helped as a nurse, Reiki practitioner, and cancer survivor. Vivi would be happy that I shared her story, which I hope illustrates how thoughts and emotions have the potential to not just heal but harm.

As I have learned more about integrative and alternative approaches to cancer treatment over the years, I wonder whether Vivi might have lived even longer had she gone to one of the Tijuana clinics. Instead of laughing at the idea as we did when Vivi returned from the hospital, I wonder why we didn't seriously research other options, especially after Vivi received the settlement from the hospital and could afford treatment. Vivi and Bailey O'Brien both had metastatic melanoma, and I can't help but wonder if Vivi would have responded to the Coley's fluids and other treatments as well as Bailey did.

Then again, I wonder whether some people rely on medical treatments too much, focusing on cancer as a disease with only physical causes and physical treatments. Some may ignore the healing power of infusing one's life with more joy, practicing forgiveness, reducing stress, and increasing social and spiritual connection—the things that appeared to have lengthened Vivi's survival.

In addition to numerous personal stories about people who attribute their recovery to psycho-spiritual changes, there is an abundance of scientific research that can explain why these factors are so important. The sciences of psychoneuroimmunology and epigenetics, as well as what is known about the physiology of stress, validate the importance of including the mind, emotions, and spirit into an individualized healing and recovery plan.

Thank you for reading my book. I leave you now with the lines of the loving-kindness meditation that is a foundation of my spiritual practice.

May you be well
May you be happy
May you be safe
May you be peaceful and at ease
May you be blessed

APPENDIX A:
Clinic Contact Information

Chapter 7

International Bio Care Hospital, Zona Rio
800-701-7345 http://www.biocarehospital.com

Bio-Medical Center (Hoxsey Clinic), Zona Rio
619-704-8442 http://www.hoxseybiomedical.com

Chapter 8

Oasis of Hope, Playas de Tijuana
888-500-4673 http://www.oasisofhope.com

Stella Maris Clinic, Zona Rio
619-405-5199 http://www.stellamaris.com

Integrative Whole Health Clinic, Zona Rio
800-910-0699 http://www.iwhclinic.com

San Diego Clinic, Zona Rio
619-804-7783 http://www.sdiegoclinic.com

Chapter 9

Baja Health and Wellness, Playas de Tijuana
866-535-8886 https://gersonplus.com

CHIPSA Hospital, Playas de Tijuana
855-624-4772 http://chipsahospital.org

St. Andrews Clinic, Playas de Tijuana
619-730-0787 http://www.standrewsclinic.com

Northern Baja Healing Center, Rosarito
715-299-5070 http://www.gersontreatment.com

Sanoviv Medical Institute, Rosarito
800-726-6848 http://www.sanoviv.com

Chapter 10

Rubio Cancer Center, Zona Rio
866-519-9960 http://rubiocancercenter.com

Hope4Cancer, Playas de Tijuana
888-544-5993 http://hope4cancer.com
Immunity Therapy Center, Zona Rio
619-870-8002 https://www.immunitytherapycenter.com

CMN Hospital, San Luis Colorado, near Yuma, Arizona
844-371-1117 http://www.cmnact.com

CIPAG/Dr. Castillo, Zona Rio
664-683-5700 (Mexico #) http://www.drcastillo.com

Europa Institute, Zona Rio
909-338-3533 http://www.europainstitute.org

Issels Immuno-Oncology, Zona Rio (inpatient) Santa Barbara, CA
(outpatient)
888-447-7357 http://www.issels.com

Angeles Functional Oncology, Zona Rio
866-668-9263 https://www.angeleshealth.com

APPENDIX B:

Alternative/Integrative Doctors/Clinics in the U.S.

MD – Medical Doctor

DO – Doctor of Osteopathy: Possesses the exact same privileges and scope of practice as MDs.

ND – Naturopathic Doctor: Possesses four years of post-graduate naturopathic medical education. Licensed in 22 states in the U.S.; scope of practice varies from state to state. Some may order laboratory testing, perform venipuncture and administer intravenous therapies, and function as family practice physicians.

ARIZONA

An Oasis of Healing, Mesa, AZ
Thomas Lodi, MD
http://www.anoasisofhealing.com

Dayspring Cancer Clinic, Scottsdale AZ
Andrew Dickens, ND; Aldemir Coelho, MD
http://www.dayspringcancerclinic.com

EuroMed Foundation, Phoenix, AZ
Frank George, DO
http://www.euro-med.us

Nature Works Best, Tempe, AZ
Coleen Huber, ND
http://www.natureworksbest.com

Partners in Integrative Cancer Therapies, Prescott, AZ
Robert J. Zieve, MD
http://www.arizonaintegrativecancer.com

Sunridge Medical Center, Scottsdale, AZ
http://www.sunridgemedical.com

CALIFORNIA
Cancer Center for Healing, Irvine, CA
Leigh Erin Connealy, MD
http://www.cancercenterforhealing.com

Issels Immuno-Oncology, Santa Barbara, CA
http://www.issels.com

Ben Johnson, MD, DO, ND, Encinitas, CA
http://www.drbenmd.com

Quantum Functional Medicine, Carlsbad, CA
Juergen Winkler, MD
http://www.qfmed.com

FLORIDA
Dayton Dandes Medical Center, Sunny Isles, FL (Miami)
Martin Dayton, MD, DO
http://www.daytondandesmedical.com

Utopia Wellness, Oldsmar, FL (near Tampa)
Carlos Garcia, MD
http://www.utopiawellness.com

GEORGIA
Center for Advanced Medicine, Johns Creek, GA (near Atlanta)
Jonathan Stegall, MD
http://www.drstegall.com

ILLINOIS
The Ayre Clinic for Contemporary Medicine, Burr Ridge, IL (near Chicago)
Thomas L. Hesselink, MD
http://www.contemporarymedicine.net

The Block Center for Integrative Cancer Treatment, Skokie, IL (near Chicago)
Keith Block, MD
http://www.blockmd.com

KANSAS
Riordan Clinic, Wichita, KS (also has locations in Hays and Kansas City, KS)
Ron Hunninghake, MD
http://www.riordanclinic.org

NEVADA
Forsythe Cancer Care Center, Reno, NV
James Forsythe, MD
http://www.drforsythe.com

The Nevada Center of Alternative and Anti-Aging Medicine, Carson City, NV
Frank Shallenberger, MD
http://www.antiagingmedicine.com/frank-shallenberger

Reno Integrative Medical Center, Reno, NV
Robert Eslinger, DO
http://www.renointegrativemedicalcenter.com

NEW YORK
Linda Isaacs, MD, New York, NY
http://www.drlindai.com (long-time partner of Dr. Nicholas Gonzalez
before his death)

Schachter Center for Complementary Medicine, Suffern NY (near New
York City)
Michael Schachter, MD
http://www.mbschachter.com

Jesse Stoff, MD, Westbury, NY (Long Island)
http://www.drstoff.com
(I know two patients who highly recommend Dr. Stoff)

NORTH CAROLINA
Center for Advanced Medicine and Clinical Research, Cornelius, NC (near
Charlotte)
Rashid Buttar, DO
http://www.drbuttar.com

Holistic Medical Clinic of the Carolinas, Wilkesboro, NC
R. Ernest Cohn, MD, ND
http://www.holisticmedclinic.com

TEXAS
Burzynski Clinic, Houston, TX
Stanislaw Burzynski, MD
http://www.burzynskiclinic.com

Kotsansis Institute, Grapevine, TX
Constantine Kotsanis, MD
http://www.kotsanisinstitute.com

VIRGINIA
Natural Horizons Wellness Centers, Fairfax, VA
Joseph Shaw Jones, MD
http://www.nhwellnesscenters.com

Resources to Locate a Functional or Integrative Medicine Doctor in the U.S.

ACAM: The American College for Advancement in Medicine has a search function to find an integrative physician by zip code and specialty. http://www.acam.org.

IFM: The Institute of Functional Medicine has a function to search for functional medicine practitioners by zip code, and in addition to MDs and DOs, also includes naturopaths, nutritionists, chiropractors, nurse practitioners, and physician assistants. https://www.ifm.org.

OncANP: The Oncology Association of Naturopathic Physicians, Inc. Has a search function to locate naturopaths who treat cancer. http://www.oncanp.org.

Orthomolecular.org: Has a directory of practitioners that offer nutritionally based therapies. Has listings in states where resources are scarce, with many that offer intravenous vitamin C. http://orthomolecular.org.

Best Answer for Cancer Foundation: Has a searchable data base of integrative physicians.

http://www.bestanswerforcancer.org.

APPENDIX C:

Common Alternative Cancer Treatments/Therapies

Information has been gathered from numerous sources to create this glossary of some of the primary therapies that are often offered in the alternative/ integrative clinics of Mexico, Germany, and for some, the U.S. as well. There are many additional therapies that may be used in the alternative/integrative clinics in Mexico, as well as those in Germany and the United States. This is a description of only those most commonly used.

Biological Dentistry

Many, if not most, doctors who treat cancer holistically believe that toxicities of the oral cavity contribute to the development of cancer and interfere with efforts to achieve lasting remission after treatment. These toxicities include the mercury and other metals present in amalgam fillings, as well as the cavitations (empty spaces) caused by root canals that may serve as a breeding ground for chronic infection and resultant inflammation. Biological dentists are specially trained to eliminate the toxicities, infection, and inflammation, and replace the metals with biologically compatible resins. Many of the clinics in Tijuana have dentists they refer patients to for the removal of root canals and replacement of amalgam fillings. The Cancer Tutor website has a lengthy and informative article about biological dentistry: https://www.cancertutor.com/biological-dentistry/.

Chelation

Chelation is an FDA-approved treatment for the removal of toxic heavy metals from the body, widely used for lead poisoning. It is performed with the chelating agent EDTA (ethylenediaminetetraacetic acid), which is an arterial cleansing agent that removes substances that congest, restrict, and impede blood flow and oxygen throughout the blood vessels. EDTA is also thought to bind with and remove the excessive free radicals that many attribute to the development and progression of cancer. Many alternative/integrative physicians believe that chelation is a very helpful detoxification treatment for those who have received chemotherapy, as many chemo drugs contain metals. Chelation may be administered intravenously or orally. The Utopia Wellness Center in Florida has an informative article on its website about the benefits of chelation for those with cancer: https://utopiawellness.com/chelation-therapy-for-cancer/.

Coffee Enemas
Coffee enemas are recommended by many alternative/integrative physicians worldwide for detoxification, pain relief, and production of the powerful antioxidant glutathione. As mentioned in chapter 1, coffee enemas have a long history of therapeutic use, and at one time they were listed in the Merck Manual, an important reference book used by conventional physicians. The late physician Nicholas Gonzalez provided a succinct explanation of why coffee enemas are beneficial in a video found on YouTube: https://www.youtube.com/watch?v=qycZ3mfmQBM.

Dendritic cell vaccines
As mentioned in chapter 2, dendritic cells are a type of white blood cell that are sometimes referred to as the sentinels or policemen of the immune system, as they notify other immune cells of the presence of malignant cells that should be eradicated. To create a dendritic cell vaccine, the patient's blood is drawn and used to create a vaccine that is specific to the patient's own cancer. It takes two or three weeks for a laboratory to culture the blood and create the vaccine, which is why most of the clinics send a patient home with the vaccine after only a dose or two is administered at the clinic. This is a simplistic description; more information about dendritic cell vaccines, and their potential to help those with cancer, can be found at: https://dendritic.info/dc-therapy/. On this website you will find information about dendritic cell

216

research and clinical trials, as well as an informative video by Dr. Edgar Engleman of Stanford University. There are many academic articles on PubMed (https://www.ncbi.nlm.nih.gov/pubmed) discussing the use of dendritic cell vaccines for cancer.

Escozine

Escozine is a trademarked product made with the venom of the blue scorpion, commonly found in Cuba and other tropical locations. There are a few articles that present research studies that have found scorpion venom to have anti-carcinogenic effects, and scorpion venoms have been used in the traditional medicine of various cultures for many years. An academic article about the anti-cancer properties of scorpion venom can be found at: https://www.ncbi.nlm.nih.gov/pubmed/24599885.

Hydrazine Sulfate

Hydrazine sulfate is a chemical compound that is thought to block a tumor from taking in glucose, slowing its growth. According to the National Cancer Institute, in some clinical trials hydrazine sulfate was reported to be helpful treating the anorexia (loss of appetite) and cachexia (wasting away) caused by cancer: https://www.cancer.gov/about-cancer/treatment/cam/patient/hydrazine-sulfate-pdq. It is not approved by the FDA as a cancer treatment. Hydrazine sulfate has also been reported to interrupt the ability of the liver to convert the lactic acid from tumors into glucose, helping to starve cancer cells.

Hyperbaric Oxygen

Hyperbaric oxygen therapy (HBOT) is a treatment that enhances the body's natural healing process, and involves inhaling 100% oxygen while in a special body chamber. Most, if not all, alternative/integrative cancer clinics offer HBOT. It is FDA approved and covered by health insurance in the United States when used to treat a variety of conditions, but is not approved to treat cancer. HBOT is a therapy that is often used in U.S.-based alternative/integrative clinics, as they are permitted to use it "off label" for indications that are not approved by the accepted standard of care for cancer. It is thought that an environment of high oxygen slows the growth of cancer and triggers apoptosis (programmed cell death). An academic article review of HBOT and its effects on cancer cells can be found at: https://www.ncbi.nlm.nih.gov/pmc/articles/PMC3510426/.

Hyperthermia

The idea that heat can treat cancer is ancient, dating back to ancient Egypt. Hyperthermia is fundamental to the treatment of cancer in alternative/integrative clinics worldwide, and is increasingly being used and studied in conventional treatment as well. As mentioned in chapter 2, cancer cells are more sensitive to the effects of high heat than normal cells, and are thought to have an impaired ability to adapt their blood circulation to the effects of high temperatures. The increased temperature weakens or kills cancer cells and makes them more vulnerable to other cancer killing therapies. Using specialized equipment, hyperthermia can be used locally for superficial tumors and as a whole body treatment for other cancers. An informative academic article that details the mechanisms in which hyperthermia is helpful for cancer therapy can be found at: https://www.ncbi.nlm.nih.gov/pmc/articles/PMC4558619/. In addition, the National Cancer Institute has an information page about hyperthermia that addresses its use and potential in cancer treatment. https://www.cancer.gov/about-cancer/treatment/types/surgery/hyperthermia-fact-sheet.

Immunotherapies

In addition to the dendritic cell vaccine described above and in chapter 2, other immunotherapies are used in some of the alternative/integrative clinics which are not FDA approved or available in the United States. Some of the physicians in the alternative/integrative clinics have particular research interest and expertise in using a variety of immunotherapies. It is beyond the scope of this book to explain the actions of every specific immunotherapy used, but all seek to enhance in some way the patient's own immune system function to eradicate cancer. These vaccines, considered experimental, include the NK/LAK vaccine, tumor-infiltrating lymphocyte vaccine, AllergoStop vaccine, Neo-Springer vaccine, and Newcastle vaccine, among others.

Infrared Saunas

Infrared saunas use radiant energy to penetrate the body's tissue to a depth of about 1.5 inches, and are believed to aid in detoxification by increasing the ability of the skin to cleanse via profuse sweating. They are also believed to increase oxygenation, improve circulation, and support immune function. Traditional saunas found in fitness centers, etc., use temperatures as high as 185 to 195 degrees Fahrenheit, which some may find intolerable for any length of time. Infrared saunas use a milder temperature of 120 to 150 degrees Fahrenheit, and the heat of infrared saunas penetrates more deeply into the body. Many people recovering from cancer purchase infrared saunas for home use. Prices start at about $1500.

Intravenous Vitamin C

Intravenous vitamin C in high doses is a standard therapy for cancer in most, if not all, alternative/integrative clinics worldwide. As mentioned in chapter 2, it is considered by some to be a nontoxic chemotherapeutic agent due to its unique actions. Recent research examined the effectiveness of vitamin C in its ability to stop the growth of cancer stem cells, and it was found to be ten times more effective than one of the experimental drugs tested alongside vitamin C. The study's lead author said that the results of the study indicate it is a promising agent for clinical trials, and as an add-on to more conventional therapies, to prevent tumor recurrence, further disease progression, and metastasis. This study also revealed that vitamin C works by inhibiting glycolysis, the process by which glucose is broken down within the cell's mitochondria and turned into energy for cancer cell proliferation. For details of this study, see: https://www.medicalnewstoday.com/articles/316334.php.

Another recent research study done at NYU Langone Health, Perlmutter Cancer Center, found that vitamin C encouraged blood cancer stem cells to die, through complex enzymatic reactions. For details of this study, see: https://www.sciencedaily.com/releases/2017/08/170817141722.htm.

IVC has been used for decades and has been found to be safe with minimal to no side effects. There are a few medical conditions that prevent the use of IVC, including certain heart and kidney conditions, as well as high iron levels, so it is important to receive this therapy by a knowledgeable doctor. For those who choose to receive conventional cancer treatment, or even for those who are in hospice care, it would be worthwhile to seek out a health care provider who offers IVC. The Riordan Clinic in Kansas is a good source of more information about the benefits of IVC: https://riordanclinic.org/what-we-do/high-dose-iv-vitamin-c/.

Laetrile

Also referred to as amygdalin or vitamin B17, laetrile is a glycoside that occurs naturally in at least one thousand different plants. To create the therapeutic compound, laetrile is extracted from the kernels of the apricot, peach, and bitter almond. As mentioned in chapter 8, no other therapy has been the subject of as much controversy as laetrile. In addition to the arguments and conflicting reports regarding its effectiveness as a cancer treatment, laetrile critics refer to it as a dangerous poison due to the presence of cyanide within the compound. Although it does contain cyanide, the most common theory about why it spares normal cells, while killing cancer cells, is due to complex enzymatic reactions that occur within the body, neutralizing the cyanide molecule. For a thirty-minute informative discussion about laetrile by Ralph Moss and Eric Merola, the producer of the film *Second Opinion: Laetrile at Sloan-Kettering*, visit https://www.youtube.com/watch?v=N5lF-rrDN3k. Another film on YouTube about laetrile, narrated and written by G. Edward Griffin, author of *World Without Cancer—The Story of Vitamin B17*, can be found at: https://www.youtube.com/watch?v=JGsSEqsGLWM.

Mistletoe

European mistletoe, mentioned in chapter 2 and often called by brand names Iscador and Helixor, is a plant that has been used for centuries to treat numerous human ailments and for over one hundred years to treat cancer in Switzerland and Germany. It has been studied extensively and is thought to act as a regulator of the immune system and have direct anti-tumor activities. It is believed to stop or slow metastasis and cause the cancer cell to revert to a more differentiated form. At least one study found that the survival time of patients treated with Iscador was 40% longer for all types of cancer. Mistletoe is used in most of the alternative/integrative clinics in Mexico and Germany, as well as in other countries where it is legal. Although it appears that many alternative/integrative clinics in the United States use it, the FDA does not allow injectable mistletoe to be imported, sold, or used, according to the National Cancer Institute, except for clinical research. A listing of doctors/clinics who use mistletoe in their practice can be found on the Believe Big website. http://believebig.org/find-a-mistletoe-doctor/#1480800356407-d6d7e491-240a. Thanks to Ivellise Page, stage IV cancer survivor and cofounder of the organization Believe Big, the early stages of developing a mistletoe clinical trial are underway at Johns Hopkins' The Sidney Kimmel Comprehensive Cancer Center, in Baltimore, Maryland. According to the Johns Hopkins website, patients are slowly being enrolled for a Phase I clinical trial, during which safety, dosage, and side effects will be assessed. For more information, see: https://www.hopkinsmedicine.org/kimmel_cancer_center/research_clinical_tr ials/clinical_trials/mistletoe.html.

Naltrexone (low-dose)

Naltrexone is an FDA-approved drug for the treatment of opioid addiction. In low doses, it has been found to boost the response of the immune system, activating the body's own natural defenses, and has been used safely for the treatment of cancer and autoimmune diseases. See: https://www.lowdosenaltrexone.org/ldn_and_cancer.htm.

Ozone Therapy

Ozone is a type of oxygen, consisting of three atoms of oxygen attached together, versus the more stable element containing two atoms of oxygen that we breathe. It is believed that cancer cells die when exposed to oxygen, due to their anaerobic nature. Ozone therapy uses a sterile system into which six to twelve ounces of blood from the body is withdrawn. The blood is saturated with oxygen (ozone), before the oxygen-rich blood is returned to the body. The benefits are believed to be increased oxygen delivery to cells, tissues, and organs, as well as an increase in blood circulation throughout the body. Ozone therapy is said to aid in detoxification, stimulate the immune system, and aid in healing external wounds. Ozone therapy has proven to be very safe and has been used in the Mexican and German alternative/integrative clinics for many years. A comprehensive resource for information on oxygen therapies can be found at: http://www.oxygenhealingtherapies.com/Medical_Ozone_Cancer.html.

PEMF

PEMFs (pulsed electromagnetic fields) are thought to reduce pain and inflammation, improve oxygenation of tissues, and improve energy, circulation, and immune function. PEMF therapy is FDA approved for bone fractures, and a form of electromagnetic therapy called Optune is FDA approved for certain brain cancers. PEMF is thought to concentrate nutrients in the tumor area and promote increased exchange by electrically opening and closing both cancerous and healthy cells. The uptake of nutrients boosts the function of the healthy cells and weakens the cancer, while the elimination of wastes detoxifies the area and promotes proper cellular metabolism. An academic article with information about the anti-cancer effects of PEMF can be found at: https://www.ncbi.nlm.nih.gov/pmc/articles/PMC5119968/.

Photodynamic Therapy

Photodynamic therapy (PDT) is a treatment that uses a typically nontoxic drug called a photosensitizer and a particular type of light. The photosensitizer is given intravenously or applied to the skin. When the photosensitizer is exposed to a specific wavelength of light, a form of oxygen is produced that kills cancer cells and, according to the American Cancer Society, may also help by destroying the blood vessels that feed the cancer cells and alerting the immune system to attack the cancer. Since the light cannot pass through more than about one-third of an inch of tissue, PDT is usually used to treat more superficial tumors. This treatment is used in conventional oncology with an FDA-approved photosensitizing agent to treat or relieve the symptoms of esophageal cancer and non-small-cell lung cancer, as well as precancerous lesions in patients with Barrett's esophagus. Side effects are reported to be mild and temporary. According to the National

Cancer Institute, clinical trials are in progress to evaluate the use of PDT for cancers of the brain, skin, prostate, cervix, and peritoneal cavity. Researchers are also trying to develop photosensitizers that are more powerful, target cancer cells more specifically, and are activated by light that can penetrate tissue and treat deeper and larger tumors. For an article about the use of photodynamic therapy at the Roswell Park Cancer Institute in New York, see: https://www.roswellpark.org/cancertalk/201702/new-way-deliver-photodynamic-therapy. Some clinics use Sonodynamic therapy, a less-studied treatment, whereby specific sensitizers are used that respond to sound, often ultrasound, rather than light.

Poly-MVA

Poly-MVA is a dietary supplement containing a blend of the mineral palladium bonded to alpha-lipoic acid, vitamins B1, B2, and B12, and other amino acids and trace minerals. It is believed to change the electrical potential of cells and facilitate metabolism within the cell. According to the developer of the supplement, Poly-MVA reduces tissue and cellular damage due to radiation, assists in promoting healthy cell integrity, protects DNA from oxidative damage, acts as an antioxidant and detoxifier, enhances white blood cell function, and supports nerve and neurotransmitter function. Physician James W. Forsythe of the Forsythe Cancer Care Center, in Nevada, is very enthusiastic about the use of Poly-MVA, and has an informative article on the clinic's website describing the supplement and his research that supports its use in cancer treatment: http://www.centurywellness.com/article-archives/233-poly-mva-new-cancer-breakthrough-for-advanced-cancer-patients.

Rife Therapy

In the 1930s the FDA and AMA discredited, harassed, and eventually shut down the work of pioneering scientist and inventor Dr. Royal Raymond Rife, who discovered that viruses and cancer cells have a unique electrical frequency. Among many other inventions, including the most powerful microscope of the era, Rife invented a device he called a frequency generator, that he claimed could kill cancer cells using certain frequencies of radio waves.

The effectiveness of the frequency generator was reported to have been tested in a 1934 trial of sixteen patients with advanced cancer at the Scripps Institute, with a designated research committee from the University of California supervising the trial. According to published reports, fourteen of the patients were declared cured after seventy days of treatment with the frequency generator by the physicians overseeing the trial, with the other two patients declared cured after an additional three weeks. Although Dr. Rife did have many supporters, his ideas were considered preposterous by most in mainstream medicine, and his treatment of cancer patients with the frequency generator was considered quackery by the medical establishment despite the positive results from the Scripps trial. When having Rife Therapy, special pads are placed on the body that deliver the electromagnetic pulse. Rife Therapy is similar to PEMF, although Rife Therapy attempts to determine and match the electromagnetic frequency of a particular cancer, whereas PEMF does not. There are many videos on YouTube describing the therapy as well as the controversy that surrounded it and Royal Raymond Rife.

Rigvir

Rigvir is an oncolytic/oncotropic virus therapy developed in Riga, Latvia, at the International Virotherapy Center. Approved by the equivalents of the FDA in Latvia, the Republic of Georgia, and Armenia, it is a therapy of increased interest worldwide, especially for melanoma. Rigvir reportedly finds and selectively infects tumor cells, then replicates in the tumor cells, destroying them. Normal, healthy cells are reported to be minimally, if at all, affected. Rigvir is said to be effective in inducing remission, improving quality of life, and improving survival. Rigvir is not FDA approved or available in the United States or Canada, although a few American and Canadian doctors have received training at the International Virotherapy Center. To my knowledge, outside of Europe, Rigvir is available at only two clinics in Tijuana, Hope4Cancer and Sanoviv, and the Freeport Family Wellness Centre in the Bahamas. Rigvir is administered as a series of injections in the buttocks or arms over approximately three years, given at intervals determined by the treating physician in an individualized treatment plan. There are not yet any clinical trials in progress in the United States. For more information visit the International Virotherapy Center: www.rigvir.com. Ralph Moss believes there is insufficient evidence of the effectiveness of Rigvir, and in his blog says that he would avoid Rigvir until proponents produce more credible documentation of its effects: http://www.ralphmossblog.com/2016/07/rigvir.html.

There is one oncolytic virus therapy for cancer that received FDA approval in 2015, however. T-VEC (Imlygic) is used for the treatment of some patients with metastatic melanoma. It must be injected directly into the tumors, typically every two weeks. It is a genetically modified virus, unlike Rigvir, which is a naturally occurring virus found in healthy people.

Stem Cell Therapy

Several alternative/integrative clinics use autologous stem cell therapy for patients with cancer. Autologous refers to the fact that the patient is the donor of the healthy stem cells, extracted via either a blood draw, removal from the bone marrow of the patient's hip bone or sternum, or from fat cells via a liposuction procedure. There are clinics in Mexico, and worldwide, that use embryonic stem cells, sometimes from animals. Some feel that using embryonic stem cells risks the transfer of viral infections or other blood-borne complications. The use of human embryonic stem cells is fraught with ethical concerns. Transplanted autologous stem cells show anti-inflammatory and immune modulating activity, which can regulate the immune system and suppress abnormal immune reactions. Essentially, a stem cell transplant provides new stem cells that can make new, healthy blood cells, stimulating natural processes to help the body fight cancer. Since chemotherapy targets rapidly dividing cells, including healthy bone marrow, stem cell transplantation is thought to aid in recovery from the immune-suppressing effects of chemotherapy. Bone marrow stem cell transplant has been used for years in conventional oncology, typically after the administration of aggressively high doses of chemotherapy that decimate the healthy stem cells within the bone marrow. For more information about bone marrow stem cell transplants, see: https://www.cancer.net/navigating-cancer-care/how-cancer-treated/bone-marrowstem-cell-transplantation/what-stem-cell-transplant-bone-marrow-transplant.

Ultraviolet Blood Irradiation

Ultraviolet blood irradiation (UBI) is a procedure that involves removing a small quantity of blood from a patient which is then exposed to ultraviolet light. The bacteria and viruses in the blood are killed by the light, creating a self-generated vaccine. When the blood is then returned to the patient, a strong immune response is created. In addition to strengthening the body's immune system against bacteria and viruses, UBI is also thought to have anti-inflammatory effects, improve circulation and tissue oxygenation, and stimulate the production of red blood cells. UBI was used in the past to treat a variety of diseases, before the discovery and development of antibiotics. With the emergence of antibiotic-resistant strains of bacteria, UBI is receiving renewed interest. An academic article about the use and benefits of UBI can be found at: https://www.ncbi.nlm.nih.gov/pmc/articles/PMC4783265/. The hospital CMN-ACT has an informative page about using UBI for cancer patients: http://www.cmnact.com/Blog/2016/November/What-is-Ultraviolet-Blood-Irradiation-UBI-and-ho.aspx.

ENDNOTES

Chapter 2

1 Anguille, S., Smits, E.L., Lion, E., van Tendeloo, V.F., & Berneman, Z.N. (2014). *Clinical use of dendritic cells for cancer therapy.* Lancet Oncology, 15(7), e257-267. doi: 10.1016/S1470-2045(13)70585-0. https://www.ncbi.nlm.nih.gov/pubmed/24872109.

2 *Duke physicians turn up heat on tumors to hasten their demise.* (2016). Duke Health News. https://corporate.dukehealth.org/news-listing/feature-duke-physicians-turn-heat-tumors-hasten-their-demise.

3 *Vitamin C and cancer: Antitumor activity of sodium ascorbate therapy.* Riordan Clinic. https://riordanclinic.org/research-study/vitamin-c-cancer-antitumor-activity-sodium-ascorbate-therapy/.

4 Fritz, H., Flower, G., Weeks, L., Cooley, K., Callachan, M., McGowan, J., … & Seely, D. (2014). *Intravenous vitamin C and cancer: A systematic review.* Integrative Cancer Therapies, 13(4), 280-300. doi: 10.1177/1534735414534463. https://www.ncbi.nlm.nih.gov/pubmed/24867961.

5 Grossarth-Maticek, R., Kiene, H., Baumgartner, S.M., & Ziegler, R. (2001). Use of Iscador, an extract of European mistletoe (Viscum album), in cancer treatment: prospective nonrandomized and randomized matched-pair studies nested within a cohort study. Alternative Therapies in Health and Medicine, 7(3), 57–66, 68–72, 74–76. https://www.ncbi.nlm.nih.gov/pubmed/11347286.

6 Ostermann, T., Raak, C., & Büssing, A. (2009). *Survival of cancer patients treated with mistletoe extract (Iscador): a systematic literature review.* BMC Cancer, 9, 451. http://doi.org/10.1186/1471-2407-9-451. See also Marvibaigi, M., Supriyanto, E., Amini, N., Abdul Majid, F. A., & Jaganathan, S. K. (2014). *Preclinical and clinical effects of mistletoe against breast cancer.* BioMed Research International, 2014. http://doi.org/10.1155/2014/785479.

7 Mistletoe extracts (PDQ®) – Health professional version. National Cancer Institute. https://www.cancer.gov/about-cancer/treatment/cam/hp/mistletoe-pdq.

8 Weber, Wendy. (2016, September 27). *Building a foundation for clinical trials of natural products.* https://nccih.nih.gov/research/blog/natural-products-clinical-trials.

9 Buhrmann, C., Kraehe, P., Lueders, C., Shayan, P., Goel, A., & Mehdi, S. (2014). *Curcumin suppresses crosstalk between colon CSC and stromal fibroblasts in the tumor microenvironment: Potential role of EMT.* PLOS ONE. https://doi.org/10.1371/journal.pone.0107514. Retrieved from http://journals.plos.org/plosone/article?id=10.1371/journal.pone.0107514.

10 Zhi, H., Ou, B., Luo, B.M., Feng, X., Wen, Y.L, & Yang, H.Y. (2007). *Comparison of ultrasound elastography, mammography and sonography in the diagnosis of solid breast lesions.* Journal of Ultrasound in Medicine, 26(6), 807–815. https://www.ncbi.nlm.nih.gov/pubmed/17526612. See also *Elastography: New cancer detection method right around the corner; Norway and France in front.* (2013). Science Daily. Retrieved November 2, 2016 from www.sciencedaily.com/releases/2013/02/130204094600.htm.

11 Faguet, Guy B. (2005). *The war on cancer: An anatomy of failure, a blueprint for the future.* (p. 120). Dordrecht, the Netherlands: Springer.

12 Ibid.

13 Mukherjee, Siddhartha. (2016, May 12). *The improvisational oncologist.* The New York Times. https://www.nytimes.com/2016/05/15/magazine/oncologist-improvisation.html.

14 Elizabeth, Erin. (2016, March 12). *Holistic doctor death series: Over 60 dead in just over a year.* Health Nut News. https://www.healthnutnews.com/recap-on-my-unintended-series-the-holistic-doctor-deaths/.

15 *Inspections, compliance, enforcement, and criminal investigations.* (2009). U.S. Food and Drug Administration. http://wayback.archive-it.org/7993/20161021235453/http://www.fda.gov/ICECI/EnforcementActions/WarningLetters/2009/default.htm.

16 *The genetics of cancer.* National Cancer Institute. https://www.cancer.gov/about-cancer/causes-prevention/genetics. (Updated May 1, 2017).

17 Moffitt researchers develop a novel cancer treatment approach based on evolutionary principals to inhibit chemo-resistance, prolong progression-free survival. (2016, February 24). Moffitt Cancer Center. https://moffitt.org/newsroom/press-release-archive/2016/moffitt-researchers-develop-a-novel-cancer-treatment-approach-based-on-evolutionary-principals-to-inhibit-chemo-resistance-prolong-progression-free-survival/.

Chapter 3

1 Kolata, Gina. (1998, May 3). *Hope in the lab: A special report; A cautious awe greets drugs that eradicate tumors in mice.* The New York Times. http://www.nytimes.com/1998/05/03/us/hope-lab-special-report-cautious-awe-greets-drugs-that-eradicate-tumors-mice.html.

2 von Eschenbach, A.C. (2003). *NCI sets goal of eliminating suffering and death due to cancer by 2015.* Journal of the National Medical Association, 95(7), 637–639. https://www.ncbi.nlm.nih.gov/pmc/articles/PMC2594648/pdf/jnma00311-0142.pdf.

3 Abola, M.V. & Prasad, V. (2016). *The use of superlatives in cancer research.* JAMA Oncology, 2(1), 139–141. doi:10.1001/jamaoncol.2015.3931.

4 Szabo, Liz. (2017, April 26). *How hype can mislead cancer patients, families.* *Kaiser Health News.* http://www.cnn.com/2017/04/26/health/hope-vs-hype-cancer-treatment-partner/index.html.

5 Miller, Sara G. (2017, January 5). *Cancer death rates fall as prevention, treatment advance.* Live Science. https://www.livescience.com/57398-cancer-death-rate-decline.html.

6 Mozes, A. (2017, January 5). *U.S. cancer death rates continue to fall.* CBS News Health Day. http://www.cbsnews.com/news/us-cancer-death-rates-continue-to-fall/.

7 Kolata, Gina. (April 23, 2009). *Advances elusive in the drive to cure cancer.* The New York Times. http://www.nytimes.com/2009/04/24/health/policy/24cancer.html?mcubz=0.

8 Cancer stat facts. National Cancer Institute Surveillance, Epidemiology, and End Results Program. https://seer.cancer.gov/statfacts/.

9 *An overview of the human genome project.* National Human Genome Research Institute. Last reviewed May 11, 2016. https://www.genome.gov/12011238/an-overview-of-the-human-genome-project/.

10 Wishart, D.S. (2015). *Is cancer a genetic disease or a metabolic disease?.* EBioMedicine, 2(6), 478-479. doi:10.1016/j.ebiom.2015.05.022.

11 Mukherjee, Siddhartha. (2010). *The emperor of all maladies: A biography of cancer.* (p. 443). New York, NY: Scribner.

12 Prasad, V. (2016). *Perspective: The precision-oncology illusion.* Nature 537, S63. doi:10.1038/537S63a.

13 Ibid.

14 Apple, Sam. (2016, May 5). *An old idea revived: Starve cancer to death.* The New York Times. https://www.nytimes.com/2016/05/15/magazine/warburg-effect-an-old-idea-revived-starve-cancer-to-death.html.

15 Ibid.

16 Howard, Jacqueline. (2017, June 2). *Hope and hype around cancer immunotherapy.* CNN. http://www.cnn.com/2017/06/02/health/immunotherapy-cancer-debate-explainer/index.html.

17 Chustecka, Zosia. (2015, June 1). New immunotherapy costing $1 million a year. Medscape. http://www.medscape.com/viewarticle/845707.

18 Seyfried, Thomas. (2016, July 15). *Cancer as a mitochondrial metabolic disease.* Epigenix Foundation. https://www.youtube.com/watch?v=PuG5XZSR4vs&t=1297s.

19 Steka, Bret. (2016, March 5). *Fighting cancer by putting tumor cells on a diet.* NPR Shots Health News. http://www.npr.org/sections/health-shots/2016/03/05/468285545/fighting-cancer-by-putting-tumor-cells-on-a-diet.

20 Hildenbrand, Gar. (1990). *How the Gerson therapy heals.* Gerson Research Organization. http://gerson-research.org/research/gerson-therapy-heals/.

21 Wishart. *Is cancer a genetic disease or a metabolic disease?.* EBioMedicine. doi:10.1016/j.ebiom.2015.05.022.

22 Apple (2016). *An old idea revived: Starve cancer to death.* https://www.nytimes.com/2016/05/15/magazine/warburg-effect-an-old-idea-revived-starve-cancer-to-death.html.

Chapter 4

1 DeVita Jr., V.T., & Chu, E. (2008). *A history of cancer chemotherapy.* American Association for Cancer Research. doi: 10.1158/0008-5472.CAN-07-6611 http://cancerres.aacrjournals.org/content/68/21/8643.

2 Morgan, G., Wardy, R., & Bartonz, M. (2004). *The contribution of cytotoxic chemotherapy to 5-year survival in adult malignancies.* Clinical Oncology, 16. 549–560. doi:10.1016/j.clon.2004.06.007.

3 Ibid.

4 Segelov, Eva. (2006, January 31). *The emperor's new clothes – can chemotherapy survive?* Australian Prescriber, 29(1), 2-3. doi: 10.18773/austprescr.2006.001 https://www.nps.org.au/australian-prescriber/articles/the-emperor-s-new-clothes-can-chemotherapy-survive.

5 Ibid.

6 Moss, Ralph W. (2008). *How effective is chemotherapy?.* International Center for Nutritional Research, Inc. http://www.icnr.com/articles/ischemotherapyeffective.html.

7 Abel, U. (1992). *Chemotherapy of advanced epithelial cancer—a critical review.* Biomedicine & Pharmacotherapy, 46(10), 439–452. https://www.ncbi.nlm.nih.gov/pubmed/1339108.

8 Faguet, Guy B. (2005). *The war on cancer: An anatomy of failure, a blueprint for the future.* (p. 120). Dordrecht, the Netherlands: Springer.

9 Ibid., p. 134.

10 Ibid., p. 182.

11 Weeks, J.C., Catalano, P.J., Cronin, A., Finkelman, M.D., Mack, J.W., Keating, N.L., & Schrag, D. (2012). *Patients' expectations about effects of chemotherapy for advanced cancer.* The New England Journal of Medicine, 367(17), 1616–1625. http://doi.org/10.1056/NEJMoa1204410.

12 Lipton, Bruce. (2015). The biology of belief: Unleashing the power of consciousness, matter and miracles. (p. 136). Hay House, Inc.

13 Fang, F., Fall, K., Mittleman, M.A., Sparén, P., Ye, W., Adami, H., & Valdimarsdóttir, U. (2012). *Suicide and cardiovascular death after a cancer diagnosis.* The New England Journal of Medicine, 366, 1310–1318. doi: 10.1056/NEJMoa1110307.

14 Lawenda, Brian D. (2016, March 16). The most important statistic you need to know. Integrative Oncology Essentials. https://integrativeoncology-essentials.com/2016/03/the-most-important-statistic-you-need-to-know/.

15 Angell, Marcia. (2004). The truth about the drug companies: How they deceive us and what to do about it. (introduction). New York, NY: Random House LLC.

16 Goldacre, Ben. (2012). *Bad pharma: How drug companies mislead doctors and harm patients.* (introduction). New York, NY: Faber and Faber, Inc.

17 Hutchinson, Courtney. (2011, September 23). *Getting big pharma to treat childhood cancers.* ABC News. http://abcnews.go.com/Health/CancerPreventionAndTreatment/big-pharma-treat-childhood-cancers/story?id=14571277.

18 Verma, R., Foster, R.E., Horgan, K., Mounsey, K., Nixon, H., Smalle, N., & Hughes, T.A. (2016). *Lymphocyte depletion and repopulation after chemotherapy for primary breast cancer.* Breast Cancer Research, 18(10). https://doi.org/10.1186/s13058-015-0669-x.

19 Mols, F., Beijers, T., Lemmens, V., ven den Hurk C.J., Vreugdenhil, G., & van de Poll-Franse, L.V. (2013). *Chemotherapy-induced neuropathy and its association with quality of life among 2- to 11-year colorectal cancer survivors: Results from the population-based PROFILES registry.* Journal of Clinical Oncology, 31(21), 2699–2707. https://www.ncbi.nlm.nih.gov/pubmed/23775951. See also Ezendam, N.P., Pijlman, B., Bhugwandass, C., Pruijt, J.F., Mols, F., Vos, M.C. Pijnenborg, J.M., & van de Poll-Franse, L.V. (2014). *Chemotherapy-induced peripheral neuropathy and its impact on health-related quality of life among ovarian cancer survivors: results from the population-based PROFILES registry.* Gynecologic Oncology, 135(3), 520–527. https://www.ncbi.nlm.nih.gov/pubmed/25281491.

20 Campbell, Katie A. (2016). The Courage Club: A Radical Guide for Audaciously Living Beyond Cancer. Washington, DC: Difference Press.

21 Barton, M.B., Gebski, V., Manderson, C., & Langlands, A.O. (1995). *Radiation therapy: Are we getting value for money?.* Clinical oncology, 7(5), 287–292. https://www.ncbi.nlm.nih.gov/pubmed/8580053.

22 Table 38: Radiation therapy following Mastectomy and Overall Survival in Stage II and III Breast Cancer. Susan G. Komen Foundation. http://ww5.komen.org/BreastCancer/Table38Radiationtherapyfollowingma stectomyandoverallsu rvivalinstageIIampIIIbreastcancer.html.

23 Relation, T., Dominici, M. & Horwitz, E.M. (2017), *Concise review: An (im)penetrable shield: How the tumor microenvironment protects cancer stem cells.* Stem Cells, 35(5), 1123–1130. doi: 10.1002/stem.2596.

24 Vinogradov, S. & Wei, X. (2012). *Cancer stem cells and drug resistance: The potential of nanomedicine.* Nanomedicine, 7(4), 597-615. doi: 10.2217/nnm.12.22.

25 Sun, Y., Campisi, J., Higano, C., Beer, T.M., Porter, P., Coleman, I., True, L., & Nelson, P. S. (2012). *Treatment-induced damage to the tumor microenvironment promotes prostate cancer therapy resistance through WNT16B.* Nature Medicine, 18(9):1359–1368.

26 Ibid.

27 *How a chemo drug can help cancer spread from the breast to the lungs.* (2017, August 7). Science Daily. https://www.sciencedaily.com/releases/2017/08/170807155401.htm.

28 Ibid.

29 Printz, C. (2012), *Radiation treatment generates therapy-resistant cancer stem cells from less aggressive breast cancer cells.* Cancer, 118, 3225. doi:10.1002/cncr.27701. http://onlinelibrary.wiley.com/doi/10.1002/cncr.27701/full.

30 Lagadec, C., Vlashi, E., Della Donna, L., Dekmezian, C., Pajonk, F. (2012). *Radiation-induced reprogramming of breast cancer cells.* Stem Cells, 30(5), 833–844. doi: 10.1002/stem.1058.

31 Cheng, J., Tian, L., Ma, J., Gong, Y., Zhang, Z., Chen, Z., Xu, B., Xiong, H., Li, C., & Huang, Q. (2015). *Dying tumor cells stimulate proliferation* of *living tumor cells* via caspase-dependent protein kinase Cδ activation in pancreatic ductal adenocarcinoma. Molecular Oncology, 9(1), 105–114. doi: 10.1016/j.molonc.2014.07.024.

32 Ng, A.K., Travis, L.B. (2008). *Subsequent malignant neoplasms in cancer survivors.* Cancer Journal, 14(6), 429–434. doi: 10.1097/PPO.0b013e31818d8779.

33 Petrow, Steven. (2012, July 16). *New cancer threat lurks long after cure.* The New York Times, Well Blog. https://well.blogs.nytimes.com/2012/07/16/new-cancer-threat-lurks-long-after-cure/?mcubz=0.

34 "What Are the Risk Factors for Myelodysplastic Syndromes?" Myelodysplastic Syndromes – Causes, Risk Factors, and Prevention, American Cancer Society, last revised July 2, 2015. https://www.cancer.org/cancer/myelodysplastic-syndrome/causes-risks-prevention/risk-factors.html.

35 *Robin Roberts' rare blood disorder: What is myelodysplastic syndrome?*. (2012, June 11). Fox News Health. http://www.foxnews.com/health/2012/06/11/robin-roberts-rare-blood-disorder-what-is-myelodysplastic-syndrome.html.

36 Hodgson D.C., Gilbert, E.S., Dores, G.M., Schonfeld, S.J., Lynch, C.F., Storm, H., ... & Travis, L.B. (2007). *Long-term solid cancer risk among 5-year survivors of Hodgkin's lymphoma.* Journal of Clinical Oncology, 25(12), 1489–1497. https://www.ncbi.nlm.nih.gov/pubmed/17372278.

37 Schaapveld, M., Aleman, B.M.P., van Eggermond, A.M., Janus, C.P.M., Krol, A.D.G., van der Maazen, R.W.M., ... & van Leeuwen, F.E. (2015). *Second cancer risk up to 40 years after treatment for Hodgkin's lymphoma.* The New England Journal of Medicine, 373, 2499–2511. http://www.nejm.org/doi/full/10.1056/NEJMoa1505949.

38 Travis, L.B., Fossa, S.D., Schonfeld S.J., McMaster, M.L., Lynch, C.F., Storm, H. ... & Gilbert, E.S. (2005). *Second cancers among 40,576 testicular cancer patients: focus on long-term survivors.* Journal of the National Cancer Institute, 97(18), 1353–1365. doi: 10.1093/jnci/dji278.

39 Travis, L.B., Ng, A.K., Allan, J.M., Pui, C., Kennedy, A.R., Xu, X.G., ... & Boice Jr., J.D. (2012). *Second malignant neoplasms and cardiovascular disease following radiotherapy.* Journal of the National Cancer Institute, 104(5), 357–370. https://www.ncbi.nlm.nih.gov/pmc/articles/PMC3295744/.

40 Grantzau, T. & Overgaard J. (2016). *Risk of second non-breast cancer among patients treated with and without postoperative radiotherapy for primary breast cancer: A systematic review and meta-analysis of population-based studies*

including 522,739 patients. Radiotherapy & Oncology, 121(3), 402–413. http://dx.doi.org/10.1016/j.radonc.2016.08.017.

41 "Side Effects of Targeted Cancer Therapy Drugs." American Cancer Society. Last revised June 6, 2016. https://www.cancer.org/treatment/treatments-and-side-effects/treatment-types/targeted-therapy/side-effects.html.

42 Fisher, B., Costantino, J.P., Wickerham, D.L., Redmond, C.K., Kavanah, M., Cronin, W.M., … & Wolmark, N. (1998). Tamoxifen for prevention of breast cancer: report of the National Surgical Adjuvant Breast and Bowel Project P-1 Study. Journal of the National Cancer Institute 90(18):1371–1388. https://www.ncbi.nlm.nih.gov/pubmed/9747868.

43 Richtel, Matt. (2016, December 3). *Immune system, unleashed by cancer therapies, can attack organs.* The New York Times. https://www.nytimes.com/2016/12/03/health/immunotherapy-cancer.html?mcubz=0.

44 Biological therapies for cancer. National Cancer Institute. https://www.cancer.gov/about-cancer/treatment/types/immunotherapy/bio-therapies-fact-sheet.

45 Baldo, B.A. (2013). *Adverse events to monoclonal antibodies used for cancer therapy: Focus on hypersensitivity responses.* Oncoimmunology, 2(10), e26333. http://doi.org/10.4161/onci.26333.

46 Weintraub, Karen. (2017, September 12). *Powerful childhood cancer treatment holds promise – and poses hazards.* Scientific American. https://www.scientificamerican.com/article/powerful-childhood-cancer-treatment-holds-promise-and-poses-hazards/.

Chapter 5

1 Ross, Casey, Blau, Max, & Sheridan, Kate. (2017, March 7). Medicine with a side of mysticism: Top hospitals promote unproven therapies. Stat News. https://www.statnews.com/2017/03/07/alternative-medicine-hospitals-promote/.

2 Garrow, J.S. (2007). How much of orthodox medicine is evidence based?. BMJ, 335(7627), 951. doi: 10.1136/bmj.39388.393970.1F. https://www.ncbi.nlm.nih.gov/pmc/articles/PMC2071976/.

3 Ullman, Dana. (2011, November 17). *How scientific is modern medicine really?*. Huffington Post. http://www.huffingtonpost.com/dana-ullman/how-scientific-is-modern_b_543158.html.

4 Newman, David H. (2009, April 2). *Believing in treatments that don't work*. The New York Times Well Blog. https://well.blogs.nytimes.com/2009/04/02/the-ideology-of-health-care./

5 Prasad, V., Vandross, A., Toomey, C., Cheung, M., Rho, J., Quinn, S., ... & Cifu, A. (2013). *A decade of reversal: An analysis of 146 contradicted medical practices*. Mayo Clinic Proceedings, 88(8). 790–798. http://dx.doi.org/10.1016/j.mayocp.2013.05.012.

6 Brawley, Otis Webb. (2012). *How we do harm: A doctor breaks ranks about being sick in America*. (p. 39). New York, NY: St. Martin's Press.

7 Goldacre, Ben. (2012). *Bad pharma: How drug companies mislead doctors and harm patients*. (introduction). New York, NY: Faber and Faber, Inc.

8 Leaf, Clifton. (2013). The truth in small doses: Why we're losing the war on cancer-and how to win it. (pp. 224–225) New York: Simon & Schuster.

9 Ibid. (p. 223).

10 Kolata, Gina & Pollack, Andrew. (2008, July 6). *Costly cancer drug offers hope, but also a dilemma.* The New York Times. http://www.nytimes.com/2008/07/06/health/06avastin.html.

11 Horovitz, Bruce & Appleby, Julie. (2017, March 20). Pharma TV ad spend promoting prescription drugs has increased 62 percent since 2012. Kaiser Health News. http://medcitynews.com/2017/03/pharma-tv-ad-spend-promoting-prescription-drugs/.

12 Swanson, Ana. (2015, February 11). *Big pharmaceutical companies are spending far more on marketing than research.* The Washington Post. https://www.washingtonpost.com/news/wonk/wp/2015/02/11/big-pharmaceutical-companies-are-spending-far-more-on-marketing-than-research/.

13 Wilson, Duff. (2010, March 31). *Pfizer gives details on payments to doctors.* The New York Times. http://www.nytimes.com/2010/04/01/business/01payments.html.

14 Johnson, S.B., Park, H.S., Gross, C.P., Yu, J.B. (2018). *Use of alternative medicine for cancer and its impact on survival.* Journal of the National Cancer Institute, 110(1). https://doi.org/10.1093/jnci/djx145.

15 Scutti, Susan. (2017, August 17). *Choosing alternative cancer therapy doubles risk of death, study says.* CNN. http://www.cnn.com/2017/08/17/health/alternative-vs-conventional-cancer-treatment-study/index.html.

16 Wark, Chris. (2017). *Study attacking alternative medicine proves little more than industry bias.* Chris Beat Cancer. https://www.chrisbeatcancer.com/study-attacking-alternative-medicine-proves-conventional-cancer-treatment-is-failing/.

17 Walsh, Bryan. (2014, May 29). *Why your doctor probably has a "Do Not Resuscitate" order.* Time Health. http://time.com/131443/why-your-doctor-probably-has-a-do-not-resuscitate-order/.

18 Lewis, C., Xun, P., & He, K. (2016). Effects of adjuvant chemotherapy on recurrence, survival, and quality of life in stage II colon cancer patients: A 24-month follow-up. Supportive Care in Cancer, 24(4), 1463–1471. https://www.ncbi.nlm.nih.gov/pubmed/26349575.

19 Turner, Kelly A. (2014). *Radical remission: Surviving cancer against all odds.* (p. 45). New York: Harper Collins.

Chapter 6

1 Schwabe, R.F., & Jobin, C. (2013). *The microbiome and cancer.* Nature Reviews Cancer, 13(11), 800–812. http://doi.org/10.1038/nrc3610.

2 Sonnenburg, E.D., Sonnenburg, J.L. (2014). Starving our microbial self: the deleterious consequences of a diet deficient in microbiota-accessible carbohydrates. Cell Metabolism, 20(5), 779–786. doi: 10.1016/j.cmet.2014.07.003.

3 Maroon, J.C., Seyfried, T.N., Donohue, J.P., & Bost, J. (2015). *The role of metabolic therapy in treating glioblastoma multiforme.* Surgical Neurology International, 6, 61. http://doi.org/10.4103/2152-7806.155259. See also Seyfried, Thomas. (2015, March 2). Cancer: A metabolic disease with metabolic solutions. The IHMC. https://www.youtube.com/watch?v=SEE-oU8_NSU&t=233s. See also Seyfried, Thomas. (2016, November 4). Cancer as a metabolic disease with Dr. Thomas Seyfried. Hyperbaric Medical Solutions. https://www.youtube.com/watch?v=dm_ob5u9FdM&t=2282s.

4 Seyfried (2016). Cancer as a metabolic disease with Dr. Thomas Seyfried. https://www.youtube.com/watch?v=dm_ob5u9FdM&t=2282s.

5 Steka, Bret. (2016, March 5). Fighting cancer by putting tumor cells on a diet. NPR Shots Health News. http://www.npr.org/sections/health-shots/2016/03/05/468285545/fighting-cancer-by-putting-tumor-cells-on-a-diet.

6 Schmidt, M., Pfetzer, N., Schwab, M., Strauss, I., & Kämmerer, U. (2011). *Effects of a ketogenic diet on the quality of life in 16 patients with advanced cancer: A pilot trial.* Nutrition & Metabolism, 8, 54. http://doi.org/10.1186/1743-7075-8-54.

7 Zuccoli, G., Marcello, N., Pisanello, A., Servadei, F., Vaccaro, S., Mukherjee, P., & Seyfried, T.N. (2010). *Metabolic management of glioblastoma multiforme using standard therapy together with a restricted ketogenic diet: Case report.* Nutrition & Metabolism, 7, 33. http://doi.org/10.1186/1743-7075-7-33.

8 Poff, A.M., Ward, N., Seyfried, T.N., Arnold, P., D'Agostino, D.P. (2015). Non-toxic metabolic management of metastatic cancer in VM mice: Novel combination of ketogenic diet, ketone supplementation, and hyperbaric oxygen therapy. PLOS ONE. https://doi.org/10.1371/journal.pone.0127407.

9 van Niekerk, G., Hattingh, S.M., & Engelbrecht, A.M. (2016). *Enhanced therapeutic efficacy in cancer patients by short-term fasting: The autophagy connection.* Frontiers in Oncology, 2016(6), 242. https://www.ncbi.nlm.nih.gov/pmc/articles/PMC5107564/. See also O'Flanagan, C.H., Smith, L.A., McDonell, S.B., & Hursting, S.D. (2017). *When less may be more: calorie restriction and response to cancer therapy.* BMC Medicine, 15, 106. https://doi.org/10.1186/s12916-017-0873-x. Retrieved from https://bmcmedicine.biomedcentral.com/articles/10.1186/s12916-017-0873-x.

10 O'Flanagan et al. (2017). *When less may be more: calorie restriction and response to cancer therapy.* https://bmcmedicine.biomedcentral.com/articles/10.1186/s12916-017-0873-x.

11 Connealy, Leigh Erin. (2017). *The cancer revolution: A groundbreaking program to reverse and prevent cancer.* (p. 56). Philadelphia, PA: Da Capo Press–Perseus Books.

12 McDougall, J. (2016). The McDougall newsletter, volume 15, issue 9. https://www.drmcdougall.com/misc/2016nl/sep/sugarcancer.htm.

13 Ibid.

14 Peiris-Pagès, M., Martinez-Outschoorn, U.E., Pestell, R.G., Sotgia, F., & Lisanti, M.P. (2016). *Cancer stem cell metabolism.* Breast Cancer Research, 18, 55. http://doi.org/10.1186/s13058-016-0712-6.

15 Goodwin, J., Neugent, M.L., Lee, S.Y., Choe, J.H., Choi, H., Jenkins, D.M.R., … & Kim, J. (2017). *The distinct metabolic phenotype of lung squamous cell carcinoma defines selective vulnerability to glycolytic inhibition.* Nature Communications, 8. doi:10.1038/ncomms15503. http://www.nature.com/articles/ncomms15503.

16 Gonzalez, Nicholas. (2013, September 10). *The ketogenic diet and cancer.* NaturalHealth465. http://www.naturalhealth465.com/cancer_part_8.html/.

17 Gerson, Dr. Max. The Gerson Institute. https://gerson.org/gerpress/dr-max-gerson/.

18 Hildenbrand, Gar. (1990). *Biological basis of the Gerson therapy: Salt and water management and tissue damage syndrome.* https://gerson.org/gerpress/wp-content/uploads/2011/08/Biological-Basis-of-the-Gerson-Therapy.pdf.

19 Palumbo, J.S., Talmage, K.E., Massari, J.V., La Jeunesse, C.M., Flick, M.J., Kombrinck, K.W., … & Degan, J.L. (2004). *Platelets and fibrin(ogen) increase metastatic potential by impeding natural killer-mediated elimination of tumor cells.* Blood, 105(1), 178–185. doi: 10.1182/blood-2004-06-2272.

20 Lipinski, B. & Egyud L.G. (2000). *Resistance of cancer cells to immune recognition and killing.* Medical Hypotheses, 54(3), 456–460. doi: 10.1054/mehy.1999.0876.

21 Gonzalez, Nicholas. (2015). *Different diets for different types* [DVD]. New York, NY: New Spring Press LLC.

22 Gonzalez, N. & Isaacs, L. (2007). *The Gonzalez therapy and cancer: A collection of case reports.* Alternative Therapies, 13, 1. http://www.alternative-therapies.com/at/web_pdfs/gonzalez1.pdf.

23 Gonzalez, Nicholas. (2017). Nutrition and the Autonomic Nervous System: The Scientific Foundations of the Gonzalez Protocol. (p. 4–6). New York, NY: New Spring Press LLC.

24 Gonzalez & Isaacs (2007). *The Gonzalez therapy and cancer.* http://www.alternative-therapies.com/at/web_pdfs/gonzalez1.pdf.

25 Schwedhelm, C., Boeing, H., Hoffmann, G., Aleksandrova, K., & Schwingshackl, L. (2016). *Effect of diet on mortality and cancer recurrence among cancer survivors: A systematic review and meta-analysis of cohort studies.* Nutrition Reviews, 74(12), 737–748. http://doi.org/10.1093/nutrit/nuw045. See also McEligot, A. J., Largent, J., Ziogas, A., Peel, D., & Anton-Culver, H. (2006). *Dietary fat, fiber, vegetable, and micronutrients are associated with overall survival in postmenopausal women diagnosed with breast cancer.* Nutrition and Cancer, 55(2), 132–40. doi: 10.1207/s15327914nc5502_3.

26 Schwingshackl, L., & Hoffmann, G. (2016). *Does a Mediterranean-type diet reduce cancer risk?.* Current Nutrition Reports, 5, 9–17. http://doi.org/10.1007/s13668-015-0141-7.

27 Inoue-Choi, M., Sinha, R., Gierach, G.L., & Ward, M.H. (2016). *Red and processed meat, nitrite, and heme iron intakes and postmenopausal breast cancer risk in the NIH-AARP Diet and Health Study.* International Journal of Cancer, 138(7), 1609–1618. http://doi.org/10.1002/ijc.29901.

28 Taunk, P., Hecht, E., & Stolzenberg-Solomon, R. (2016). *Are meat and heme iron intake associated with pancreatic cancer? Results from the NIH-AARP Diet and Health Cohort.* International Journal of Cancer, 138(9), 2172–2189. http://doi.org/10.1002/ijc.29964.

29 Ibid. See also Bastide, N., Pierre, H.F., Corpet, D. (2011). *Heme iron from meat and risk of colorectal cancer: A meta-analysis and a review of the mechanisms involved.* Cancer Prevention Research, 4(2), 177–184. doi: 10.1158/1940-6207.CAPR-10-0113.

30 Taunk et al. (2016). *Are meat and heme iron intake associated with pancreatic cancer?* http://doi.org/10.1002/ijc.29964. See also Lam, T.K., Rotunno, M., Ryan, B.M., Pesatori, A.C., Bertazzi, P.A., Spitz, M., … Landi, M.T. (2014). *Heme-related gene expression signatures of meat intakes in lung cancer tissues.* Molecular Carcinogenesis, 53(7), 548–556. http://doi.org/10.1002/mc.22006.

31 Fonseca-Nunes, A., Jakszyn, P., & Agudo, A. (2014). *Iron and cancer risk—A systematic review and meta-analysis of the epidemiological evidence.* Cancer Epidemiology, Biomarkers & Prevention, 23(1), 12–31. doi: 10.1158/1055-9965.EPI-13-0733.

32 Cavuoto, P. & Fenech, M.F. (2012). *A review of methionine dependency and the role of methionine restriction in cancer growth control and life-span extension.* Cancer Treatment Reviews, 38(6), 726-36. doi: 10.1016/j.ctrv.2012.01.004. See also Durando, X., Thivat, E., Gimbergues, P., Cellarier, E., Abrial, C., Dib, M., … & Chollet, P. (2008). *Methionine dependency of cancer cells: A new therapeutic approach?.* Bulletin du Cancer, 95(1), 69–76. doi: 10.1684/bdc.2008.0550. See also Cellarier, E., Durando, X., Vasson, M.P., Farges, M.C., Demiden, A., Maurizis, J.C., … & Chollet, P. (2003). *Methionine dependency and cancer treatment.* Cancer Treatment Reviews, 29(6), 489–499. http://dx.doi.org/10.1016/S0305-7372(03)00118-X.

33 Levine, M.E., Suarez, J.A., Brandhorst, S., Balasubramanian, P., Cheng, C., Madia, F., … Longo, V.D. (2014). *Low protein intake is associated with a major reduction in IGF-1, cancer, and overall mortality in the 65 and younger but not older population.* Cell Metabolism, 19(3), 407–417. http://dx.doi.org/10.1016/j.cmet.2014.02.006.

34 Jenkins, P. J., Mukherjee, A., Shalet, S.M. (2006). *Does growth hormone cause cancer?* Clinical Endocrinology, 64(2):115–121. doi: 10.1111/j.1365-2265.2005.02404.x. See also Yu, H., Rohan, T. (2000). *Role of the insulin-like growth factor family in cancer development and progression.* Journal of the National Cancer Institute, 92(18), 1472–1489. https://doi.org/10.1093/jnci/92.18.1472. See also Key, T.J. (2011). *Diet, insulin-like growth factor-1 and cancer risk.* Proceedings of the Nutrition Society, 70(3), 385–388. doi: 10.1017/S0029665111000127. See also Nimptsch, K. & Pischon, T. (2016). *Obesity biomarkers, metabolism and risk of cancer: An epidemiological perspective.* Recent Results in Cancer Research, 208, 199–217. doi: 10.1007/978-3-319-42542-9_11.

35 Sinha, R., Cross, A.J., Graubard, B.I., Leitzmann, M.F., & Schatzkin, A. (2009). *Meat intake and mortality: A prospective study of over half a million people.* Archives of Internal Medicine, 169(6), 562–571. http://doi.org/10.1001/archinternmed.2009.6.

36 IARC monographs evaluate consumption of red meat and processed meat. (2015, October 26). World Health Organization, International Agency for Research on Cancer. https://www.iarc.fr/en/media-centre/pr/2015/pdfs/pr240_E.pdf.

37 Adams, L.S., Phung, S., Yee, N., Seeram, N.P., Li, L., & Chen, S. (2010). *Blueberry phytochemicals inhibit growth and metastatic potential of MDA-MB-231 breast cancer cells through modulation of the phosphatidylinositol 3-kinase pathway.* Cancer Research, 70(9), 3594–3605. http://doi.org/10.1158/0008-5472.CAN-09-3565.

38 Ouhtit, A., Gaur, R.L., Abdraboh, M., Ireland, S.K., Rao, P.N., Raj, S.G., … Raj, M.H. (2013). *Simultaneous inhibition of cell-cycle, proliferation, survival, metastatic pathways and induction of apoptosis in breast cancer cells by a phytochemical super-cocktail: Genes that underpin its mode of action.* Journal of Cancer, 4(9), 703–715. http://doi.org/10.7150/jca.7235.

39 Thomas, R., Williams, M., Sharma, H., Chaudry, A., & Bellamy, P. (2014). *A double-blind, placebo-controlled randomised trial evaluating the*

effect of a polyphenol-rich whole food supplement on PSA progression in men with prostate cancer – the UK NCRN Pomi-T study. Prostate Cancer and Prostatic Diseases, 17(2), 180–186. http://doi.org/10.1038/pcan.2014.6.

40 Li, William Li. (2014, April 8). *Can we eat to starve cancer?.* TED-Ed. https://www.youtube.com/watch?v=OjkzfeJz660. See also Li, W.W., Li, V.W., Hutnik, M., & Chiou, A.S. (2012). Tumor angiogenesis *as a target for dietary cancer prevention.* Journal of Oncology, 2012. http://doi.org/10.1155/2012/879623.

41 Li, W.W et al. (2012). *Tumor angiogenesis as a target for dietary cancer prevention.* http://doi.org/10.1155/2012/879623.

42 Khan, N., Adhami, V.M., & Mukhtar, H. (2008). *Apoptsis by dietary agents for prevention and treatment of cancer.* Biochemical Pharmacology, 76(11), 1333–1339. http://doi.org/10.1016/j.bcp.2008.07.015.

43 Moselhy J., Srinivasan S., Ankem M.K., & Damodaran C. (2015). *Natural products that target cancer stem cells.* Anticancer Research, 35(11), 5773–5788. https://www.ncbi.nlm.nih.gov/pubmed/26503998.

44 Ibid.

45 Anand, P., Kunnumakara, A.B., Sundaram, C., Harikumar, K.B., Tharakan, S.T., Lai, O.S., … Aggarwal, B.B. (2008). *Cancer is a preventable disease that requires major lifestyle changes.* Pharmaceutical Research, 25(9), 2097–2116. http://doi.org/10.1007/s11095-008-9661-9.

46 Demark-Wahnefried, W., Rogers, L.Q., Alfano, C.M., Thomson, C.A., Courneya, K.S., Meyerhardt, J.A., … & Ligibel, J.A. (2015). *Practical clinical interventions for diet, physical activity, and weight control in cancer survivors.* CA: A Cancer Journal for Clinicians, 65(3), 167–189. doi:10.3322/caac.21265. https://www.ncbi.nlm.nih.gov/pubmed/25683894.

47 Telekes, A., Hegedus, M., Chae, C.H., & Vékey K. (2009). *Avemar (wheat germ extract) in cancer prevention and treatment.* Nutrition and Cancer, 61(6):891–899. doi: 10.1080/01635580903285114.

Chapter 8

1 Moss, R.W. (2005). *Patient perspectives: Tijuana cancer clinics in the post-NAFTA era.* Integrative Cancer Therapies, 4(1), 65–86. https://www.ncbi.nlm.nih.gov/pubmed/15695477.

2 Hess, David J. (1999). *Evaluating Alternative Cancer Therapies.* (p. 15). New Brunswick, NJ: Rutgers University Press.

Chapter 11

1 Overview of the SEER Program. National Cancer Institute, Surveillance, Epidemiology, and End Results Program. https://seer.cancer.gov/about/overview.html.

2 Gonzalez, N., Isaacs, L. (2015). *Why meaningful statistics cannot be generated from a private practice.* Alternative Therapies, 21(2), 11–15. http://www.alternative-therapies.com/openaccess/ATHM_21_2_Gonzalez.pdf.

3 Ellison, Ayla. (2016, January 13). *Average cost per inpatient day across 50 states.* Becker's Hospital CFO Report. http://www.beckershospitalreview.com/finance/average-cost-per-inpatient-day-across-50-states.

4 *Protection from high medical costs.* HealthCare.gov.
https://www.healthcare.gov/why-coverage-is-important/protection-from-high-medical-costs/.

5 *Cancer prevalence and cost of care projections, annualized mean net costs of care.* National Cancer Institute.
https://costprojections.cancer.gov/annual.costs.html.

6 Glover, Lacie. (2015, July 1). *Oncologists worry about rising costs of cancer treatment.* U.S. News and World Report. http://health.usnews.com/health-news/patient-advice/articles/2015/07/01/oncologists-worry-about-rising-costs-of-cancer-treatment.

7 *Placebo effect and lessons for the physician-patient relationship.* (2013, September 19). *ScienceDaily.*
https://www.sciencedaily.com/releases/2013/09/130919201241.htm.

8 Ellis, Rehema. (2006, September 21). *Cancer docs profit from chemotherapy drugs.* NBC News.
http://www.nbcnews.com/id/14944098/ns/nbc_nightly_news_with_brian_williams/t/cancer-docs-profit-chemotherapy-drugs.

9 Pearl, Robert. (2014, August 7). *Are oncologists recommending the best treatments for patients?.* Forbes.
https://www.forbes.com/sites/robertpearl/2014/08/07/are-oncologists-recommending-the-best-treatments-for-patients/2/#2259047328aa.

10 *Payments linked to higher odds of doctors prescribing certain cancer drugs.* (2017, June 1). University of North Carolina Lineberger Cancer Center. http://unclineberger.org/news/payments-linked-to-higher-odds.

ACKNOWLEDGMENTS

I would like to thank, first and foremost, the many patients and companions of patients whom I met in Tijuana, who were willing to share their story and insights with me. In particular, I would like to express my appreciation to the patients whom I referred to as Grace, Joy, and Hope in the book—you know who you are, and I pray for your continued healing and well-being.

Many thanks go to Bailey O'Brien, who was willing to relay her story to me in great detail by phone, edited the draft of her chapter to ensure accuracy, served as a beta reader, and allowed me to publish her story. Also many thanks to Shannon Knight, for her enthusiastic and kind support, for being willing to share her story in the foreword, and for her other contributions to the book. There were other former patients, or family members of former patients, of the Tijuana clinics who also generously shared their stories with me. Special thanks to Marie Carlson, Claudia, Maebell Beard, Janet, and Peggy.

I would also like to thank the doctors who welcomed my visit to their clinic, and were generous with their time and knowledge. If I knew then what I know now, I would have had far more questions for you! Special thanks to physicians Gilberto Alvarez, Jose A. Henriquez, Filiberto Muñoz, and Dan Rogers. Thanks to physician Edgar Payan of CMN-ACT, for taking the time to meet with me on Skype, and sharing his knowledge and insights with me. Thanks to Gar and Christeene Hildenbrand, who were willing to meet with me and share some of their vast knowledge from years of involvement with cancer treatment in Tijuana. A thank you to Robin Willis R.N. who made me feel so welcome at the Bio-Medical Center, and was so enthusiastic and supportive of my project.

To my developmental editor, the "book shaman" Melanie Bates, many

249

thanks for your support, expertise, and strong belief that I could complete this project. Many thanks to my friend and cheerleader Meredith, who not only provided insightful feedback and editing but unwavering support and encouragement. Thanks to all my friends for their support and belief in me, especially Sha Chang, cancer researcher and science mentor, who continually challenged me, and Brenda Willie, who served as a beta reader and provided invaluable support, encouragement, and feedback. Thanks to Phil Ives, who provided meticulous proofreading. Finally, many thanks go to my copy editor, Siobhan Gallagher, for her generous dedication to my book and enthusiasm for the subject matter. How I found a professional editor whose mother, now 84, happened to have received successful alternative cancer treatment for Stage IV cancer (with Dr. Rubio in Tijuana and Dr. Burzynski in Houston), twenty years ago can only be explained by serendipity, intuition, or divine intervention.

ABOUT THE AUTHOR

Katey Hansen lives in rural North Carolina with her border collie/hound mix Gracie. She is a registered nurse and is a certified cancer coach through the Center for Advancement in Cancer Education. She is also a life coach, trained by Martha Beck, Inc., and a certified Kripalu yoga teacher and Reiki Master/Teacher. When not writing, consulting, and researching, Katey loves spending as much time as possible in nature, growing vegetables in her organic garden, hiking in the forest with friends, and visiting rivers, lakes, and the ocean, whenever possible.

Katey is a holistic cancer educator and recovery consultant, and provides phone/Skype sessions for those who have been diagnosed with cancer as well as for those who wish to minimize the chance of recurrence after treatment. Katey helps people with cancer develop individualized healing/recovery plans that include body, emotions, mind, and spirit. She does not give medical advice or prescribe treatment, and always encourages people with cancer to have the support of a trusted and qualified doctor.

Katey can be contacted at katey@kateyhansen.com, or through her website, http://www.kateyhansen.com.

Made in the USA
San Bernardino, CA
07 April 2018